Essential nMRCGP® CSA Preparation and Practice Cases

Essential nMRCGP® CSA Preparation and Practice Cases

RHONA KNIGHT

MB BS, MA (Med Ed), FRCGP

Portfolio GP

Programme Director,

East Midlands Healthcare Workforce Deanery

MRCGP CSA Examiner

Foreword by

PROFESSOR SIMON GREGORY

FRCGP

Postgraduate Dean, NHS East of

England Multi Professional Deanery (formerly GP Dean,

East Midlands Healthcare Workforce Deanery)

GP

Radcliffe Publishing

Oxford • New York

Radcliffe Publishing Ltd
18 Marcham Road
Abingdon
Oxon OX14 1AA
United Kingdom

www.radcliffe-oxford.com
Electronic catalogue and worldwide online ordering facility.

British Library Cataloguing in Publication Data
A catalogue record for this book is available from the British Library.

ISBN-13: 978 1 84619 406 1

The paper used for the text pages of this book is FSC certified. FSC (The Forest Stewardship Council) is an international network to promote responsible management of the world's forests.

Mixed Sources
Product group from well-managed forests and other controlled sources
www.fsc.org Cert no. SGS-COC-2482
© 1996 Forest Stewardship Council

Typeset by Pindar NZ, Auckland, New Zealand
Printed and bound by TJI Digital, Padstow, Cornwall, UK

Contents

Foreword   vii

Preface   ix

About the author   xi

Section 1   Preparing for the CSA examination   1

1   The CSA exam   3

2   Consultation skills and the CSA   8

3   Preparing for the CSA   18

4   Meet the team: reflections on preparing for and taking the CSA   24

5   The curriculum   33

6   Writing your own cases   39

7   Marking cases and giving feedback   49

8   CSA case example 1   52

9   CSA case example 2   58

Section 2   Practice CSA cases   65

10   Robert Davies by Deborah Webb   67

11   John Bradford by Hannah Kundu   72

12   Eva Peterson by Shamit Kalla   78

13   Jane Doe by Himanshu Shekhar   83

14   Melissa Smith by Dave Sharma   89

15   Bradley Dillon by Shiloh Jacintha Jonnalagadda   93

16   Frank Spencer by Mark Shaffu   97

17   Jack West by Vicky Taylor   102

18   Lucy Waters by Kafayat Lee   107

19   Aisha Makda by Keshdip Hayer   112

20   Mukul Bhatt by Uma Mahalingappa   117

21   John Maddison by Caroline Taylor-Walker   124

22   John Griffin by Krishna Pabbaraju   129

Section 3   The next steps   **135**

23   Reflections on the process   137

24   Life beyond CSA Land   141

Index   143

Foreword

It has long been recognised that assessment drives learning. Each of us, if we are to be honest, will recognise that at times in our careers our study has been focused on what we thought the examiners would ask of us, rather than mastery of the field. The corollary of this is that ideally examiners wish to test knowledge, skills and attitudes; competencies in the chosen field not the ability to pass examinations. Reality is that the examiners examine surrogates of normal performance, examination conditions being far from normal, and candidates focus on passing the examination. This is perhaps inevitable especially in a high-stakes examination.

The new membership examination of the Royal College of General Practitioners (nMRCGP) was developed to meet the standards required by the Postgraduate Medical Education and Training Board (PMETB). It is already widely regarded as one of the best medical assessments. With GP Specialty training being too short at only three years, the nMRCGP is inevitably an exit examination. Thus in addition to the high cost of putting on and therefore of sitting the examination, the summative nature puts excessive pressure on the future GP as they approach the end of their training. There is a plethora of books, DVDs and courses capitalising on the exam and perhaps on the fears of the candidates. Rhona Knight's book is different. Rhona is a passionate and compassionate educator with a strong sense of natural justice, and also a long-standing MRCGP examiner. She has developed an approach to understanding and preparing for the Clinical Skills Assessment (CSA) that is already tried, tested and proven. An approach that will enhance the candidate's ability as a GP at the same time as preparing them for the CSA.

Rhona valiantly took on the challenge of supporting a group of GP Specialty Registrars that had started their training before the advent of the new GP curriculum and the nMRCGP, and found themselves now facing different challenges than they had expected and prepared for, the 'transition trainees'. Her approach, focusing on developing these bright young doctors as consummate GPs whilst addressing their need to pass the MRCGP, resulted in the model of preparing for the CSA that she and her 'transition team' share in this book. In this book she shares with the reader a tool that can use the assessment to drive professionalism and deep learning, not the usual pre-exam superficial learning, and she does so ethically, respecting the integrity of the CSA. Her 'feet on the ground' style and approach is accessible and the overview of consultation models and 'reflection trigger list' are useful in their own right. Using the case-writing approach candidates will not only build upon their own surgeries and knowledge whilst preparing for an exam, they will also be preparing for their careers as GPs.

The transition team of 13 trainees/candidates share their stories, their exam impressions and the cases they developed. Their generosity in so doing is typical of the many wonderful trainees that make up the young blood of our profession and I thank and congratulate them. The journey through CSA land that awaits will at times be as scary as Alice's adventures in Wonderland would surely have been. But just as Lewis Carroll's book is a childhood favourite, Rhona Knight's is sure to be a comfort and a favourite. We all wish you success in the CSA/nMRCGP and welcome you to our profession.

Professor Simon Gregory FRCGP
Postgraduate Dean, NHS East of England Multi Professional Deanery
(formerly GP Dean, East Midlands Healthcare Workforce Deanery)
GP
November 2009

Preface

An adventure in CSA land

As I run down the platform at Victoria Station, I am reminded of the White Rabbit in Lewis Carroll's *Alice's Adventures in Wonderland*, 'Oh dear! Oh dear! I shall be too late!'[1] It's a Saturday – Thameslink is closed and the engineering works on the underground have made No 1 Croydon seem a long way away. I look at my watch again.

I am then reminded of the many GP registrars, the Clinical Skills Assessment (CSA) examination candidates, who, very like Alice following the White Rabbit, will be following in my footsteps. They may not be falling down a rabbit hole, but they will be rising up in a long lift and entering the very different world of No 1 Croydon. It won't be Wonderland. It is CSA land.

When Alice arrived in Wonderland she was initially a normal size human being, but after a drink from a bottle saying 'DRINK ME', she tells us 'What a curious feeling! I must be shutting up like a telescope.'[2] In CSA land, a similar feeling can happen. While GP registrars in the real world are of normal size, and seen by their patients as doctors with expertise, able to meet the needs of their patients who come with a variety of problems that they hope the doctor can address, in CSA land it is the doctor who faces the unknown, and is being assessed while facing it. The doctor no longer has the power in the consultation. It is the 'patient' and the observing examiner. The patient has the power of knowledge of his problem, his thoughts and what he wants. The examiner has the power to pass or fail.

The aim of this book is to provide those taking the CSA exam with the antidote to the bottle that says 'DRINK ME' and provide instead a piece of cake that says 'EAT ME'. For after all, soon Alice's 'eye fell on a little glass box that was lying under the table: she opened it, and found in it a very small cake, on which the words "EAT ME" were beautifully marked in currants. "Well, I'll eat it," said Alice, "and if it makes me larger, I can reach the key."'[3] And make her grow it did. '"Curiouser and curiouser . . . now I'm opening out like the largest telescope that ever was! Good-bye, feet!"'[4]

While I hope this book keeps your feet on the ground and visible, I also hope that it will make you feel more in control of your performance in the CSA and increase your chances of passing.

This book has been made possible by the large amount of time I have spent working with role players and simulators in a variety of teaching situations, both undergraduate and postgraduate. This has given me a great insight into role play assessment and case writing generally. Thanks go particularly to the simulators in the Leicester area, especially Michele Gutteridge and Peter Worrall. I am also very indebted to Anne de la Croix, who was able to provide evidence of the impact of simulation on the power dynamics of the consultation, in her presentation at the annual conference of the Association for the Study of Medical Education, held in Leicester in 2008.

It has been good to use all of this experience in both writing and assuring cases for the CSA, a role I have performed since the inception of the new exam. Leaving this part of my examining portfolio in April 2009 has made the writing of this book possible, although I do still continue as a CSA examiner.

This book contains no actual CSA cases. None have been written or adapted from CSA cases. Instead, I have adapted the model I use for writing cases in the undergraduate context and have used the wonderful source of all cases, everyday clinical experience, to develop the examples contained here. This has been added to by using a teacher's most valuable resource, the learners, which you will see demonstrated as you go through the book. In this I am thankful to the GP training programme members who have been involved since the idea for this book was conceived.

I wish to formally acknowledge and thank the Royal College of General Practitioners for allowing me to use information from the college website. This has all been reproduced with the permission of the Royal College of General Practitioners, and the reference details are given in the relevant sections of the book. I am also grateful to my colleague programme directors, Pete Wells and Mike Davies, for their comments on the final draft. All remaining errors, however, are mine. I am also indebted to my husband, Chris Knight, for the tireless way he has gone through each new version of the manuscript pointing out areas that needed clarification and tidying up, and to my three children for their support and tolerance.

I hope you, the reader, will find this book useful as you prepare for the CSA exam and independent practice. I wish you well.

Rhona Knight
November 2009

References

1 Carroll L. *Alice in Wonderland and Through the Looking Glass.* London: Pan Books; 1947. p. 12.
2 Ibid. p. 17.
3 Ibid. p. 18.
4 Ibid. p. 20.

About the author

Dr Rhona Knight is a portfolio GP working in inner city Leicester. She has been involved in medical education for many years, and is currently a Programme Director and MRCGP Clinical Skills Assessment Examiner. She is also a Senior Clinical Educator at the University of Leicester, and is involved in training simulated patients and role players. One of her interests is enabling GP registrars to prepare for independent practice, while at the same time preparing for and passing the exams needed to complete training.

Preparing for the CSA examination

The CSA exam

'Do you mean that you think you can find out the answer to it?' said the March Hare.

'Exactly so,' said Alice.

'Then you should say what you mean,' the March Hare went on.

'I do,' Alice hastily replied; 'at least – at least I mean what I say – that's the same thing, you know.'

(Alice's Adventures in Wonderland, p. 73)

The exam

The Clinical Skills Assessment (CSA) is a high stakes, expensive examination taken towards the end of General Practice training. It is not a typical tick-box Objective Structured Clinical Examination (OSCE), but neither is it a traditional simulated surgery. Instead it is an exam that aims to be 'an assessment of a doctor's ability to integrate and apply clinical, professional, communication and practical skills appropriate for general practice'.[1] It takes a global perspective, moving beyond pure knowledge and basic competency to the application of knowledge, assessing more holistically what the doctor can do.

General Practice is complex. It has a curriculum which, when printed out, can be weighed by the kilogram, and yet even the curriculum does not define all that one needs to know and be able to do as a General Practitioner (GP). As GPs we never 'know it all'. We are always identifying new learning needs. The CSA takes all of this complexity on board, and 'tests a doctor's abilities to gather information and apply learned understanding of disease processes and person-centred care appropriately in a standardised context, making evidence-based decisions, and communicating effectively with patients and colleagues'.[2]

The exam takes place in a building in Croydon that resembles an old three-penny bit: No 1 Croydon, just outside East Croydon train station. This tall building, known by some as the 'Tower of Terror', has three of its floors, the 18th, 19th and 20th, fitted out as a bespoke assessment centre, with rooms like GP surgeries situated around the circumference of the building, each with a view overlooking the Croydon area. Each morning and each afternoon over the exam period, GP Specialty training Registrars (GPStRs), the exam candidates, arrive at No 1 Croydon. They are directed to a plenary session, where the process is explained. They then move to an assessment room on one of the three floors, where they will be met by a list of the 'patients' that they are about to see, with their relevant medical records. They will then proceed to consult with

13 'patients', the surgery being broken up by a coffee break of about 20 minutes. Of the 13 cases seen, one is a pilot case and is not included in the final mark. The cases may include home visits and telephone calls, and possibly seeing another member of the primary healthcare team, for example a nurse.

What is being assessed?

It is important to note that this is not a normal surgery. Instead, the candidate is presented with a series of cases devised to assess learning outcomes as defined in the GP curriculum. Each series of 12 cases aims to cover a representative part of the overall curriculum.

This includes:[3]

▶ data gathering and interpretation
▶ management
▶ co-morbidity and health promotion
▶ person-centred approach
▶ professional attitude
▶ technical skills.

This means that candidates will need to obtain the necessary information from the notes, take an appropriate history, perform a skilful focused examination, make a suitable choice of investigations, and interpret all the information obtained. This is just what GPs do on a day-to-day basis. Candidates also need to be able to recognise and manage common medical conditions met in General Practice, often in the context of co-morbidities. Not knowing how to recognise and manage carpal tunnel syndrome is not ideal. However, identifying and working with more acceptable gaps in knowledge, for example the inheritability of rare genetic diseases, are important skills that may also need to be demonstrated.

The process of decision-making is central to the consultation, and varies from patient to patient. While the default is that of a shared decision-making process, more paternalistic approaches can be appropriate on occasion. The art of General Practice is flexibility – addressing the need of the individual patient in front of you. This, along with the ability to promote the shared decision-making process by giving information to the patient in an understandable way, are areas the CSA seeks to assess. As GPs we need to do all of this in a professional and ethical way.

The cases

In choosing the selection of cases for a CSA 'surgery', several things are borne in mind.[4] The cases seen should cover a selection of different body systems, e.g. neurological, cardiovascular and respiratory. These are then assessed in a variety of contexts:

▶ acute illness
▶ chronic illness
▶ undifferentiated illness
▶ psychological and social aspects of illness
▶ preventative and lifestyle issues.

This ensures that the assessment covers a representative sample of the curriculum.

Although the list of 'patients' seen on different CSA days are unlikely to be the same, for fairness it is intended that each candidate should be presented with a similar spectrum of cases, although quite possibly in different system areas. These should be at a similar level of difficulty. Updated information on this process is held on the RCGP website,[5] a compulsory reference for anyone taking the CSA.

Take a moment to think

It is worth at this point thinking what kind of cases may 'turn up' in the exam. What type of patients have you seen in the last week, whose stories could be adapted for examination purposes? I work in the inner city. In my last surgery, about a third of the patients I saw did not speak good English, and many of these needed an interpreter. I saw a young child with diarrhoea and vomiting, several patients with skin rashes necessitating a full examination of their skin, a patient needing a vaginal examination, and a father, who had phoned a colleague the previous day wondering if his daughter was pregnant, but not wanting us to let on to his daughter that he had phoned ahead. Which of these cases could be examined in a CSA exam?

Unfortunately, interpreted consultations are, practically, difficult to assess in a high stakes exam. At least one of the candidates is likely to speak the language. This is one of the failings of the exam as I see it. Many of the registrars I teach spend a significant part of their time consulting in languages other than English, and yet this exam only assesses English-speaking General Practice, which is not the same as UK General Practice. Time may tell whether this will change.

Young children and babies could not be used in this assessment, due to the laws relating to children working. It is therefore necessary to use proxy consulters, for example a mum consulting about her child's eczema, or behaviour, or constipation . . . The list could go on.

Patient examination is another interesting area. While it should be assessed, the CSA has limitations not seen in workplace-based assessment. A full skin examination, in the context of a whole CSA consultation, would be a struggle to fit into 10 minutes, but it is also difficult to simulate widespread psoriasis and eczema. However, an assessment of a patient with knee pain, palpitations or a cough is easier as long as there are no abnormal findings to be detected. When it comes to intimate examinations, most of us would consider a vaginal examination on a 'real' simulated patient inappropriate.

The CSA can test the *choice* of examination, the *ability* to examine and the *interpretation* of examination findings. So, for example, you may *choose* to examine a patient with palpitations. You may go on to demonstrate your *ability* in this area. You will then need to *interpret* the actual findings, or those given to you on a card by the examiner. For some cases you will probably *not* be expected to examine. You will indicate to the patient that you wish to examine them, and in the light of what you say you wish to examine you will be given the examination findings on a card by the examiner, for you to then *interpret* and use.

If we return to my last surgery, the only consultation that seems like it could be adapted for the CSA is the one with the daughter/father/pregnancy dilemma. However, this would need two role players, not the usual one, increasing the costs of an already very expensive exam. It is therefore, I suggest, a scenario which is highly unlikely to appear in the CSA.

The message

The CSA, while reliable, cannot test real-world General Practice, only aspects of it. Therefore, while consulting in General Practice will help you prepare for the exam, targeted preparation is also ideal. This is what this book is intended to enable you to do. The fact that the 'patients' seen in the CSA are role players also needs to be considered. In General Practice, the 'power' lies with the doctor. In the CSA the 'power' lies with the role player. It is not a doctor–patient relationship. It is a role-player–doctor relationship, which is a very different entity, and which needs to be understood and worked with. It is hoped that this book will give you insight into the different power dynamics, so that you can use this to help you pass the exam.

Box 1.1 presents a practical exercise to help you to start thinking about what sort of cases might and might not turn up in the CSA exam. Box 1.2 presents a worked example of the questions of Box 1.1.

BOX 1.1 Practical exercise reflecting and analysing possible CSA cases

Practical exercise

1   Look through your surgeries for the past week. What were the main problems the patients presented with?

2   Could any of these be assessed in the CSA?

3   Write down a list of possible cases that could be adapted for the exam. (Do not note down identifiable data.)

4   Now look at the curriculum statements that might be relevant to the case.

5   Identify relevant learning outcomes in these curriculum statements that could be tested.

6   What might the examiner be looking for?

7   Identify your learning needs.

BOX 1.2 Worked example of a possible CSA case

Worked example

1 Home visit to 76-year-old lady with hearing problems. Housebound with good social support.
2 Yes. Could be adapted for exam. Could be done as a home visit.
3 Home visit to a 76-year-old lady with hearing problems.
4 Care of Older Adults.
5 Learning outcomes[6] could be:
   • appropriate communication skills for counselling, teaching and treating patients, their families and carers, recognising the difficulties of communicating with older patients including the slower tempo, possible unreliability and the evidence of third parties
   • skills in history taking, physical examination and use of ancillary tests to diagnose conditions presented by patients in primary care
   • understanding of the management of the conditions and problems commonly associated with old age such as Parkinson's Disease, falls, gait disorders, stroke, confusion, etc.
6 Examiner looking for good history taking, ENT examination that will help diagnosis (tuning forks), negotiated management plan. Need to consider patient's hearing problem throughout this process.
7 Need to revise tuning fork tests.

References

1 Royal College of General Practitioners. *Clinical Skills Assessment*. Available at: www.rcgp-curriculum.org.uk/nmrcgp/csa.aspx (accessed 13 May 2009).
2 Royal College of General Practitioners. *The Clinical Skills Assessment, September 2008*. Available at: www.rcgp-curriculum.org.uk/Files/Exams_CSA_presentation_2008-2009.ppt Slide 3 (accessed 3 November 2009).
3 Royal College of General Practitioners. *The Clinical Skills Assessment, September 2008*. Available at: www.rcgp-curriculum.org.uk/Files/Exams_CSA_presentation_2008-2009.ppt Slide 13 (accessed 3 November 2009).
4 Royal College of General Practitioners. *The Clinical Skills Assessment, September 2008*. Available at: www.rcgp-curriculum.org.uk/Files/Exams_CSA_presentation_2008-2009.ppt Slide 14 (accessed 3 November 2009).
5 The College website is available at: www.rcgp.org.uk (accessed 8 July 2009). The CSA homepage is available at: www.rcgp-curriculum.org.uk/nmrcgp/csa.aspx (accessed 8 July 2009).
6 Royal College of General Practitioners. *Care of Older Adults*. Curriculum Statement 9; version 1.1, Feb 2009. Available at: www.rcgp-curriculum.org.uk/PDF/curr_9_Care_of_Older_Adults_v1_1_feb09.pdf (accessed 8th July 2009).

2

Consultation skills and the CSA

'This here young lady,' said the Gryphon, 'she wants for to know your history, she do.'

'I'll tell it her,' said the Mock Turtle in a deep, hollow tone: 'sit down, both of you, and don't speak a word till I've finished.'

So they sat down, and nobody spoke for some minutes. Alice thought to herself, 'I don't see how he can ever finish, if he doesn't begin.' But she waited patiently.

'Once,' said the Mock Turtle at last, with a deep sigh, 'I was a real Turtle.'

These words were followed by a very long silence, broken only by an occasional exclamation of 'Hjckrrh!' from the Gryphon, and the constant heavy sobbing of the Mock Turtle. Alice was very nearly getting up and saying, 'Thank you, sir, for your interesting story,' but she could not help thinking there must be more to come, so she sat still and said nothing.

(*Alice's Adventures in Wonderland*, p. 100)

Heinz 57

Consultation skill models are a bit like 'Heinz 57' – they come in many varieties. Which of these varieties you are taught depends upon which training programme you are attached to in the country. In a similar way, undergraduate teaching of consultation models varies from university to university, although most start off with what has been called the 'hospital model'. In this model, students ask patients about the following areas:

▶ presenting complaint
▶ history of present complaint
▶ past medical history
▶ drug history
▶ family history
▶ social history
▶ psychiatric history
▶ menstrual history
▶ systems review.

This form of history taking, an inductive history, is lengthy and is often finished with little engagement of the brain. The diagnostic process is not dynamic, and is completed, often unsuccessfully, by synthesising the information once the boxes have all been ticked, at the end of the consultation. It tends very much toward the 'medical' model of disease. Once in clinical practice, whether in primary or secondary care, history taking changes and becomes guided more by the patient and by the likelihood of disease and illness. The diagnostic process is ongoing, and continues throughout the consultation. With more experience, pattern recognition is increasingly embedded within this process.

It is into this arena that an increasing number of consultation models are stepping, many with overlapping themes, some with more unique perspectives. The key 'varieties' that I believe are most applicable for GP training, looked at over an historical timeline, are described below.

Key consultation models

The Doctor, his Patient and the Illness (Balint 1957).[1] This is a classic text, which I thoroughly enjoyed reading as a registrar. It introduces many concepts, all of which are as relevant to consultations today as they were back in 1957. Its main aim is to look at the key themes in the doctor–patient relationship that lead to adverse outcomes for both doctor and patient. It explores the emotional responses of doctors in the consultation and introduces the idea of the doctor as 'drug'. Other concepts covered include the 'apostolic' function of the doctor and the idea of no one taking responsibility, the 'collusion of anonymity'.

Transactional analysis (Berne 1964).[2] Although this is not specifically a medical text, Eric Berne's accessible book looks at how people interact with each other. Transactional analysis examines 'transactions' between individuals and provides some interesting insights, particularly when reflecting on a consultation or watching a video. It can also be quite useful in working out what is going on in relationships at home and at work. Berne describes three states of functioning; that of parent, adult and child. Those we interact with can also adopt each of these three states. Put simply, as an example – although Berne adds more complexity to this – if my eldest child wants to have an adult-to-adult conversation with me, and I want to have an adult-to-adult conversation with him, all is well. However, if I decide to go into parent mode and wish to put him in child mode, while he wants to function in an adult-to-adult mode, I wish to function in a parent-to-child mode and we have what is called a 'crossed transaction'. All does not go well.

The Future General Practitioner (RCGP 1972)[3] explores different dimensions of the consultation, including Ideas, Concerns and Expectations (ICE) and the bio-psychosocial model.

The exceptional potential in each primary care consultation (Stott and Davis 1979)[4] looks at the four tasks of the consultation, which, in the light of the Quality and Outcomes Framework (QOF),[5] seems to have made a bit of a comeback, as the doctor's agenda once again rears its head. The four tasks comprise:
- management of presenting complaint
- modification of help-seeking behaviour
- management of continuing problems
- opportunistic health promotion.

Six Category Intervention Analysis (Heron 1975),[6] is a favourite of mine, as I grew up on it in my own Vocational Training Scheme (VTS) in Guildford. In this model, different interventions in the consultation are described. The first three are classed as doctor-centred interventions, and the latter three as patient-centred. The interventions are:

▶ prescriptive interventions
▶ informative interventions
▶ confronting interventions
▶ catalytic interventions
▶ supportive interventions
▶ cathartic interventions.

Six phases of the consultation (Byrne and Long 1976).[7] As a 14-year-old I remember going to see my GP, now a well-known name in postgraduate medical education, and being asked if I would mind him recording the consultation on an audiotape. On discovering the work of Byrne and Long 10 years later, I did wonder whether my consultation was one of those studied and used to identify the six phases of the consultation. These phases, as described by Byrne and Long, are:

▶ the doctor establishing a relationship
▶ the doctor discovering the reason for attendance
▶ the doctor conducting a verbal and/or physical examination
▶ the doctor and patient considering the problem
▶ discussing management
▶ terminating the consultation.

Helman's folk model (Helman 1981).[8] Cecil Helman, a medical anthropologist, explores the differing perspectives of both doctor and patient: disease and illness. He identifies the 'what' and 'why' questions that patients ask about their illness. These questions are:

▶ what has happened?
▶ why has it happened?
▶ why has it happened to me?
▶ why has it happened now?
▶ what would happen if nothing were done about it?
▶ what should I do about it or whom should I consult for further help?

The Anxious Patient (Bendix 1982).[9] This small, easy-to-read green book that you can usually get from the hospital library explores the therapeutic dialogue, giving hints on how to conduct the interview. These hints promote listening to the patient and include: repeating the patient's last words to encourage them to continue talking and the advice that when you don't know what to say, you should stay quiet. The use of repeating what has been said and summary is also explored.

Disease-illness model (McWhinney 1986).[10] In 1986, Ian McWhinney, building on previous work with colleagues,[11] posited a change to a 'transformed clinical method'.[12] In this proposed move from the 'traditional method', doctors were to seek to understand their patient's perspective, and try to enter their patient's world to understand their experience of illness. This entailed using a patient-centred method as opposed to a doctor-centred method in consultations. Along with Levenstein and others,[13] this was explored further, looking in more detail at the two parallel agendas in the consultation: that of the patient and that of the doctor. The doctor's agenda relates mainly to the disease process, symptoms and signs, investigations and differential diagnosis. The patient's agenda relates to ICE, thoughts, fears, feelings and an understanding of the experience of the illness. For a satisfactory consultation, both agendas need to be considered. This focus on different agendas is developed further in Middleton's *The Team Guide to Communication*.[14]

The seven tasks of the consultation (Pendleton *et al.* 1984).[15] This book was very influential in the development of the old Membership of the Royal College of General Practitioners (MRCGP) video exam, and one can still see many signs of this in the Consultation Observation Tool (COT) assessment on the NHS e-portfolio.[16] Although the original book has now been updated,[17] the seven tasks of the consultation remain and seem as relevant today as in 1984. As GPs we need to:

▶ define the reason for the patient's attendance
▶ consider other problems
▶ choose an appropriate action
▶ achieve a shared understanding
▶ involve the patient in the management plan
▶ use time and resources appropriately
▶ establish and maintain an ongoing relationship with the patient.

This model acknowledges the patient's agenda, and the importance of identifying the patient's reason for attending by identifying their ICE and the effect of the problem on the patient's life.

The Inner Consultation (Neighbour 1987).[18] The next variety of model to arrive was Roger Neighbour's Inner Consultation, which has now become a classic. Neighbour describes the two heads the doctor needs to use in a consultation: the responder and the organiser. He moves on to describe five tasks of the consultation: connecting; summarising; handing over; safety netting and housekeeping, using the aide memoire of a hand of four fingers and a thumb. As a younger doctor, I found the introduction to housekeeping – looking after myself between consultations – a revelation, which is still of ongoing benefit in an increasingly pressurised job. Another concept, that of gift-wrapping management plans, has seen my management plans become more bespoke to the individual in front of me, increasing, I hope, concordance. A good read.

Calgary-Cambridge (1998).[19] As a teacher, this is probably my favourite model, and it is worth all registrars looking at the 71 different skills described, although the whole book can be seen by many as a bit heavy and detailed. This approach divides the consultation into five main areas:

▶ initiating the consultation

- gathering information
- building the relationship and facilitating the patient's involvement
- explanation and planning
- closing the consultation.

Explicit concepts and skills such as agenda setting, chunking and checking, contracting and signposting are described, which many registrars find useful in managing increasingly complex consultations. These are not covered so well, if at all, in other models. The area that is lacking, and this is lacking in all the models that I have described so far, is that of problem solving. How do we make diagnoses in the consultation, and how do we develop skills to do this better?

This is where the **Leicester Assessment Package (LAP)**[20] fits in. The LAP is a tool that has been adapted and used for teaching both undergraduates and postgraduates in Leicester, as well as further afield and even internationally. The postgraduate tool[21] looks at seven areas of the consultation: history taking; examination; management; problem solving; relationship with patients; anticipatory care and record keeping. It defines key competences needed in a consultation and identifies strategies to help doctors demonstrate those competences. It describes the process of problem solving, using the hypothetico-deductive model, which includes raising and testing diagnostic hypotheses. For me, it blends the 'white coat' and 'cardigan' skills needed to be a good GP. As doctors we need to be clinically competent, 'white coat', but with the communication skills, 'cardigan', to get the information needed to make a diagnosis, to share our thoughts with the patient, and to develop an evidence-based, negotiated management plan, optimising concordance and patient well-being. This particular model, which I only discovered in 2004, can help doctors structure consultations in both primary and secondary care. Its approach to the cognitive aspect of the consultation helps ensure doctors don't miss possible diagnoses, and its slant on problem solving and 'engaged brains' throughout the consultation makes for efficient use of time. Its strategies for looking at the 'cardigan' aspects of consulting are useful for those who find these areas more challenging. It is the foundational tool that I use to teach GP registrars, and much of the LAP can be implicitly seen in the approaches to consultation analysis and case writing used in this book.

Which model for the CSA?

The first thing to say is that if you have a good, well-developed, personalised consultation model that meets the needs of your patients, it is very likely to meet the needs of the CSA. The CSA assesses the 'white coat' and the 'cardigan' skills of medicine. It currently does this in three domain areas (*see* Box 2.1). Domains 1 and 2 are very 'white coat' skills, and domain 3 is the 'cardigan'. Both are needed to consult and both will be needed to pass the CSA.

BOX 2.1 The three CSA domains[22]

1 Data-gathering, technical and assessment skills

Gathering and using data for clinical judgement, choice of examination, investigations and their interpretation. Demonstrating proficiency in performing physical examinations and using diagnostic and therapeutic instruments. (*Blueprint: Problem-solving skills, Technical Skills*)

2 Clinical management skills

Recognition and management of common medical conditions in primary care. Demonstrating a structured and flexible approach to decision-making. Demonstrating the ability to deal with multiple complaints and co-morbidity. Demonstrating the ability to promote a positive approach to health. (*Blueprint: Primary care management, Comprehensive approach*)

3 Interpersonal skills

Demonstrating the use of recognised communication techniques to understand the patient's illness experience and develop a shared approach to managing problems. Practising ethically with respect for equality and diversity, in line with the accepted codes of professional conduct. (*Blueprint: Person-centred approach, Attitudinal aspects*)

The following tools aim to help you focus on the areas that typically make for a good consultation. Figure 2.1 is a flow diagram bringing out some of the key aspects from the many different consultation models described above. It is a simple approach to help you to think about the structure of your consultations, and consider whether you need to add or change anything. It can be used as it is for simple consultations, and adapted for more complex ones, for example a patient with multiple problems. Box 2.2 gives a 'reflection trigger list' that you can use after a consultation to reflect on what you achieved, in order to identify any areas that could be developed further next time.

Please don't use any model as a checklist. If you are sitting the CSA, remember you are a skilled clinician. *Don't* try to just 'tick boxes' or second guess what the examiner is looking for. Just try to consult as a good doctor, responding to the patient in a patient-centred way, using both your consultation and communication skills.

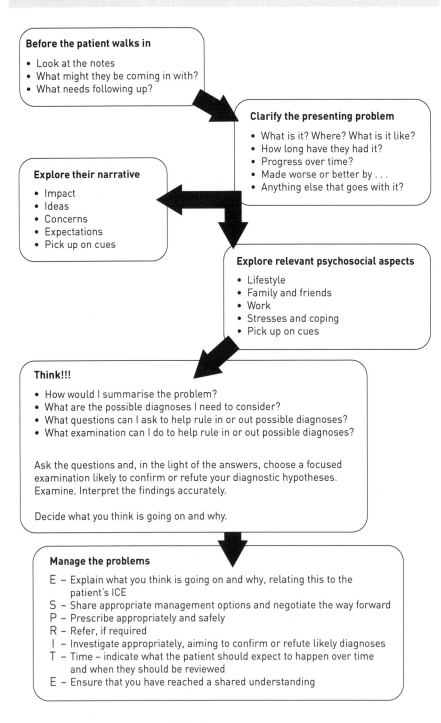

Before the patient walks in

- Look at the notes
- What might they be coming in with?
- What needs following up?

Clarify the presenting problem

- What is it? Where? What is it like?
- How long have they had it?
- Progress over time?
- Made worse or better by . . .
- Anything else that goes with it?

Explore their narrative

- Impact
- Ideas
- Concerns
- Expectations
- Pick up on cues

Explore relevant psychosocial aspects

- Lifestyle
- Family and friends
- Work
- Stresses and coping
- Pick up on cues

Think!!!

- How would I summarise the problem?
- What are the possible diagnoses I need to consider?
- What questions can I ask to help rule in or out possible diagnoses?
- What examination can I do to help rule in or out possible diagnoses?

Ask the questions and, in the light of the answers, choose a focused examination likely to confirm or refute your diagnostic hypotheses. Examine. Interpret the findings accurately.

Decide what you think is going on and why.

Manage the problems

E – Explain what you think is going on and why, relating this to the patient's ICE
S – Share appropriate management options and negotiate the way forward
P – Prescribe appropriately and safely
R – Refer, if required
I – Investigate appropriately, aiming to confirm or refute likely diagnoses
T – Time – indicate what the patient should expect to happen over time and when they should be reviewed
E – Ensure that you have reached a shared understanding

FIGURE 2.1 Key aspects of various consultation models

BOX 2.2 Reflection trigger list

Reflection trigger list

- *Did you clarify the problem?*
  — Can you summarise the key features?

  — Can you summarise the key issues?

  — Can you place the problem in context?

- *Did you explore the patient's narrative?*
  — Did you know what they were thinking about the problem?

  — Did you know how it was impacting on them and their family?

  — Did you know what they understood about what's going on?

  — Did you know what they were hoping to get out of seeing you?

- *Did you examine appropriately?*
  — Did you know what examination was needed?

  — Did you know how to do it?

  — Did it confirm or refute your possible diagnosis?

  — Did you need to examine anything else?

- *Management*
  — Did you explain effectively what you thought was going on and why?

  — Did you explicitly link this explanation with their narrative?

  — Did you give appropriate advice on self-help?

  — Did you choose the right investigations?

  — Are there any other investigations you would like to have done? Why?

  — Are there any you think were unnecessary? Why?

  — Did you prescribe properly?

  — Did you consider interactions and side effects?

  — Did you explain these to the patient?

— Did you need to refer?

— Did you refer to the right person?

— Did you know how to refer?

— What advice did you give the patient about follow-up? Why?

— How do you know this was correct for this patient?

— Did you negotiate the management plan?

— What aspects were negotiated?

— Was the management plan evidence-based? On what evidence was it based?

— Was the patient happy with the management plan?

— Did they understand it?

- *Interpersonal skills*
  — Did you behave in a professional way?

  — Did you demonstrate empathy and respect?

  — What did you discover about the psychosocial aspects of the story?

  — Did you need to know more?

  — How could you have found this out?

  — What cues did you notice?

  — What cues did you pick up on?

  — What cues did you miss?

  — How did you achieve concordance?

  — What tensions were present?

  — How well did you deal with them?

References

1   Balint M. *The Doctor, his Patient and the Illness*. 2nd ed. London: Pitman; 1964. 1st ed. 1957.

2   Berne E. *Games People Play: the psychology of human relations*. Harmondsworth: Penguin; 1964.

3   Royal College of General Practitioners. *The Future General Practitioner – Learning and Teaching*. London: RCGP; 1972.

4   Stott NCH, Davis RH. The exceptional potential in each primary care consultation. *J R Coll Gen Pract*. 1979; **29**: 201–5.

5   Further information on QOF is available at: www.dh.gov.uk/en/Healthcare/ Primarycare/Primarycarecontracting/QOF/index.htm (accessed 8 July 2009).

6   Heron J. *Six Category Intervention Analysis*. Guildford: Human Potential Resource Project, University of Surrey; 1975.

7   Byrne PS, Long BEL. *Doctors Talking to Patients*. London: HMSO; 1976.

8   Helman CG. Disease versus illness in General Practice. *J R Coll Gen Pract*. 1981; **31**: 548–52.

9   Bendix T. *The Anxious Patient: the therapeutic dialogue in clinical practice*. Edinburgh: Churchill Livingstone; 1982.

10 McWhinney IR. Are we on the brink of a major transformation of clinical method? *CMAJ*. 1986; **135**(8): 873–8.

11 McCracken EC, Stewart MA, Brown JB, *et al*. Patient-centred care: the family practice model. *Can Fam Physician*. 1983; **29**: 2313–6.

12 McWhinney, op. cit.

13 Levenstein JH, McCracken EC, McWhinney IR, *et al*. The patient-centred clinical method. 1. A model for the doctor-patient interaction in family medicine. *Fam Pract*. 1986; **3**(1): 24–30.

14 Middleton J. *The Team Guide to Communication*. Oxford: Radcliffe Medical Press; 2000.

15 Pendelton D, Schofield T, Tate P, *et al*. *The Consultation: an approach to learning and teaching*. Oxford: Oxford University Press; 1984.

16 Available at: www.nhseportfolios.org/Anon/AboutUs.aspx (accessed 8 July 2009).

17 Pendleton D, Schofield T, Tate P, *et al*. *The New Consultation*. Oxford: Oxford University Press; 2003.

18 Neighbour R. *The Inner Consultation*. Lancaster: MTP Press; 1987.

19 Silverman J, Kurtz S, Draper J. *Skills for Communicating with Patients*. Oxford: Radcliffe Medical Press; 1998.

20 Fraser RC. *Assessment of Consultation Competence. The Leicester Assessment Package*. 2nd ed. Macclesfield: Glaxo Medical Fellowship; 1994. Fraser RC. Assessing and enhancing consultation performance. In: Fraser RC, editor. *Clinical Method: a general practice approach*. 3rd ed. Oxford: Butterworth Heinemann; 1999.

21 Available at: www.gp-training.net/training/tools/lap.htm (accessed May 14 2009).

22 Royal College of General Practitioners. *The Clinical Skills Assessment, September 2008*. Available at: www.rcgp-curriculum.org.uk/Files/Exams_CSA_presentation_ 2008-2009.ppt Slide 9 (accessed 3 November 2009).

3

Preparing for the CSA

'Would you tell me, please, which way I ought to go from here?'
 'That depends a good deal on where you want to get to,' said the Cat.
 'I don't much care where –' said Alice.
 'Then it doesn't matter which way you go,' said the Cat.
 '– so long as I get somewhere,' Alice added as an explanation.
 'Oh, you're sure to do that,' said the Cat, 'if you only walk long enough.'

(Alice's Adventures in Wonderland, p. 68)

As I said in Chapter 2, many of you reading this will already have a personalised well-developed consultation model that meets the needs of your patients. If this is true, it is very likely to meet the needs of the CSA. It is really important that you don't ruin the dynamic of each individual doctor–patient relationship you have by reverting to a tick-box approach to the consultation that you think will get you through the CSA. The consultation is not a linear progression – it is complex, and needs to flow out of the doctor–patient relationship. It is about who you are as a doctor and who the patient is with whom you are interacting. It's a bit like being part of a *pas de deux* in a ballet. There are certain movements and skills that can be used, but they vary in both appropriateness and timing, each and every dance being unique.

The flow diagram in Figure 2.1 gave an idea of the possible structure of a consultation. However, this needs to be interpreted loosely. If a patient comes in oozing cues out of every part of their being and you dive mechanistically into clarifying the presenting problem, that will inevitably impact on how the patient perceives you and will adversely affect the potential of the consultation. The first part of the consultation can be a bit like a sorting office, where letters are directed into the relevant mail boxes, according to their destination. In the same way with patients, we can take and explore the information they give, fitting that into our own little filing system, identifying the gaps we need to fill in order to complete our understanding when the opportunity arises. However this does not give licence for complete disorder in the consultation. Examining or managing the problem before you have even clarified the nature of the problem is almost invariably doomed to failure.

In this chapter I will outline eight steps of preparation for the CSA. I will then go on to look at the setting up and running of a learning set, focused on preparing specifically for the CSA. This is something I have encouraged my GP registrars to do, and they have found it helpful. In the rest of the book, you will meet a team of registrars who were part of a Transition Training Programme in the East Midlands Healthcare Workforce Deanery, running from February to July 2009, and you will see some of the resources that they have prepared. These resources should help in setting up and running a learning set, focusing and directing your time effectively.

Eight steps to happiness

Step 1: observe yourself

The first step is to start watching your own video consultations, ideally with your trainer. What are your strengths? What are your weaknesses? Can you pick up on cues? Are you organised? Can you problem solve? What knowledge gaps can you identify? What examination skills need improving? Spend a lot of time doing this. It is the one opportunity in your career for getting one-to-one feedback on your consultations on a regular basis. Grab the opportunity with both hands!

Step 2: reflect, read and try out new consultation tools

Choose one of the consultation books and read it. Maybe don't start with Balint, but Pendleton or Neighbour are each an easy read. What skills could you try out? Try them. Video a few more consultations and have a few joint surgeries. What are your strengths? What areas do you need to work on? How do you identify the patient's concerns? Might there be other ways? What cues do you tend to miss? How could you be more sensitive to them? How do you deal with patients with lists? What might you do to try to manage them better?

You can then repeat this process over the training time you spend in practice, increasing the number of consultation skills you can use effectively in the consultation. It is a bit like an apprentice learning to use all the tools needed by the master craftsman. The more tools that can be used well, the better equipped the apprentice is for dealing with each and every consultation, no matter how complex or challenging.

Step 3: use your training programme

If your day release programme includes consultation skills training, do it and enjoy it, but unless it is specifically a CSA training session, don't turn it into one. I have seen one too many registrars undermine their development in consultation skills by turning wonderful learning opportunities into 'a possible CSA case' and losing out on the many other things that could have been explored. Use every opportunity you can to learn from others who are training with you. Some of them will have skills you will want to learn, copy and use. In the same way, others will learn from you. Remember, consulting in front of colleagues is often harder than consulting in front of a stranger, so learning in this way can help prevent some of the performance anxiety in the actual CSA exam.

Step 4: find out about the exam

Once your CSA is about 4 months away, start preparing properly for the exam. How do you do this?
▶ Make sure you know what is required.
▶ Find out the latest information on the RCGP website.

Step 5: set up a learning set
- Get together a learning set of about five or six people.
- Try to make sure that your learning set is varied in makeup and background.
- Arrange to meet on a regular basis and decide how you are going to run the learning set.
- Learn together and from each other.

A learning set is a way of helping people to learn from each other and to learn together. An ideal learning set has about six members. In this context it enables those present to prepare, experience and observe simulated consultations, reflecting on the process, learning from the process and planning how to do it differently next time. This then leads on to trying it out again. In doing this, Kolb's learning cycle,[1] an adapted version of which is in Figure 3.1, is 'recycled' time and again.

The relationships in the learning set allow for supported learning, and as the group gets to know each other well, the level of challenge may well increase. The diversity of the group will encourage a sharing of strengths and identification of and help for areas of weakness. Action planning at the end of each session allows for ongoing learning and division of labour. Rather than all six people looking up six sets of the latest evidence on the management of gout, each group member can look up and evaluate a different set of evidence and can then bring and present their findings to the group.

The group does not need to be facilitated, but a rolling leadership role can be useful. Group rules are a necessary element, but while these may be bespoke, they can usually be translated from the training programme small group work already being attended.

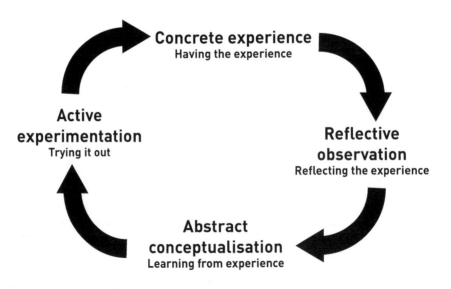

FIGURE 3.1 David Kolb's learning cycle

Step 6: use the learning set

Real consultations with real patients are a very different entity to consultations with role players. In the former, the power and medical knowledge lies with the doctor, who controls the consultation and how it flows, and can impart and apply their expertise to the situation in hand. Doctors begin and end the consultation, ask the majority of the questions, have access to the broad knowledge base required to make a diagnosis, and identify possible management options.

In role plays, the role player has the power and the knowledge. The role player knows the role and where it can go. Followed cues will lead to a greater understanding for the doctor, but the role player already knows them. If the doctor suggests certain options, the role player knows what they themselves will choose. If the doctor suggests blood tests, the role player may be primed to ask what and why, knowing how they will react to the answers.

In the CSA, this power differential is magnified. Not only does the candidate have to play a role (after all this is a performance and not a real consultation), but an examiner is watching, and the high stakes of the exam can also add increasing pressure and a feeling of further disempowerment. After all, the failing candidate at best is left £1400 worse off and at worst is left without a job or career in General Practice.

It is here we see the benefit of a learning set. In this set, those taking the CSA can get used to:
 performing
 having their performance assessed
 performing with a role player who has more 'power' and knowledge than they do
 making a huge mistake and still carrying on, not letting it affect the rest of the performance.

Step 7: structure the learning

Write a case. The first thing that is needed is to get an awareness of what makes a good CSA case. The best way to do this is for each member of the group to write one. Ideally, ensure that each member chooses a different curriculum statement and try to write cases for patients of different ages, backgrounds and presentations. A guide to how to do this will be found in Chapter 6.

Meet as a group and run a mini-surgery. The idea is that each person role plays the case he has written. The person who is to be the candidate goes out of the room while the case writer shares with the group the case and the marking schedule, indicating what he is looking for. The candidate then comes back in and the role player/case writer goes out and 'becomes' the patient. A 10-minute consultation starts. Observers mark the case.

Depending on the size of the group, two or three 'candidates' can wait outside the 'consulting room', and consult with the same case. While this may mean 10 or 20 minutes' dead time for those waiting to consult, it does mean that one case can be used for several doctors, and those observing can pick up different approaches to dealing with the same patient.

Give feedback. Feedback is tailored to the needs of the learner and the nature of the group. I find this works well with a written feedback sheet completed by everyone watching. On it, two strengths and two areas to work on are identified.

The role player/case writer feeds back the patient's perspective.

Discuss and identify learning needs. The case is then discussed as a group, and learning needs arising from it are identified.

Divide the work. The ensuing research needed to address these learning needs is then divided amongst those present, who will bring their findings back to the next session. It is often most useful to volunteer to find out and present the area you are least knowledgeable about. There is nothing quite like teaching something to help you remember it.

Six such consultations can be fitted into a two and a half hour session, meaning everyone gets to observe, be a patient and be a doctor. At the end of the session, action plans can be decided upon, work allocated and planning for the next session started. Running such sessions on a weekly or two-weekly basis enables ongoing learning. Sessions can be varied and if time is pressurised some of the CSA books on the market provide ready-made cases that can be adapted. Several cases written by registrars in the Transition GP programme are found in Section 2 of this book. These cases were written for a CSA training day and in their original form were quite variable in their content and accuracy, yet all were used beneficially as a learning tool. It is important to remember that cases do not have to be perfect to be used, or to direct learning, as they are not being used for assessment purposes. In this book, however, the cases have been tidied up and added to by the author. The Transition team member who did the initial work-up is identified in each of the relevant chapters. You can read a bit about each of them and how they prepared for the exam in Chapter 4.

Step 8: nurture each other

The CSA exam is an exam that helps grant admittance to being a Member of the Royal College of General Practitioners. General Practice is a caring profession, and is one in which teamwork is central. Working as a team in preparation for the CSA allows you to develop skills in nurturing and caring for each other, accepting and working with each other's foibles and idiosyncrasies, which, under the stress of exam pressure, can become more apparent.

We know that International Medical Graduates (IMG) and European Union (EU) graduates are statistically more likely to fail the CSA exam. In learning sets that contain a mix of UK and European graduates, along with IMGs, UK graduates have the opportunity to learn vast amounts from the broadened perspective of non-UK graduates. UK graduates in turn can help non-UK graduates adapt to an exam that may be culturally very different to their past, and often present, clinical experience.

One of the registrars in the area in which I work, who spoke five languages as well as English, spent 70% of his time *not* consulting in English. In a deanery ST3 Diversity study day in 2008, it was discovered that 20% of the ST3 registrars present spent over 20% of their consultation time using languages other than English. These doctors seem even more disadvantaged when it comes to the CSA, and mixed learning sets of UK and non-UK trained doctors may be a way to help to address this implicit disadvantage, while at the same time increasing cultural understanding.

As a programme director, it has been good to see learning sets support and nurture each other. From my perspective, it has helped people get through the exam who would otherwise have struggled, while at the same time helping those from less diverse backgrounds improve their understanding of the wide variety of patients they will come into contact with.

Reference

1   Kolb DA. *Experiential Learning: experience as the source of learning and development*. Englewood Cliffs, NJ: Prentice Hall; 1984.

4

Meet the team: reflections on preparing for and taking the CSA

'Who are you?' said the Caterpillar.

This was not an encouraging opening for a conversation. Alice replied, rather shyly, 'I – I hardly know, sir, just at present – at least I know who I was when I got up this morning, but I think I must have been changed several times since then.'

(Alice's Adventures in Wonderland, p. 48)

The team who have helped put these resources together were all on the Transition Programme of the East Midlands Health Care Workforce Deanery, running from February to July 2009. Most of the Programme members were due to finish in July 2009. This group had typically done six months in General Practice, followed by two years in hospital medicine, completing their final six months of GP training at the end of the programme. They had one opportunity of doing the CSA while in General Practice, the May sitting of 2009, after only three months in practice. Two members actually took and passed the CSA while still in hospital posts.

The team you are about to meet were a sub-group of the Transition Programme, and were involved in an additional day of CSA training, aiming to help set up learning sets to use and develop resources and tools for CSA preparation. Before the day, each person wrote a case. On the day, the group was divided into learning sets and the training process was demonstrated. Each person played the doctor in at least three observed consultations. Each person also played at least three different patients. Everyone marked each other's performances.

In no particular order, you will now meet the team. Each of them has contributed one of the cases to be found in Section 2. They all took the CSA in May 2009 and as you meet them they are awaiting their results. You will not only find out more about their own situation, but also how they prepared for the exam and their subsequent reflections on how they found it.

Deborah Webb

Deborah is 28 and qualified from Leicester University in 2004. She is married and expecting her first child, sitting the CSA exam while six months pregnant.

She sees herself as being very lucky, having done a variety of jobs in her training relevant to General Practice. She was one of the doctors on the pilot F2 programme and got tremendous experience in Genito-Urinary Medicine (GUM) and Chemical Pathology as well as an additional Medicine post. Her other jobs included Urology, Surgery, Medicine, Accident and Emergency (A&E), Obstetrics and Gynaecology (O&G), Psychiatry and 16 months of General Practice. She hopes to be a part-time GP initially, whilst bringing up a family.

Reflecting on the exam

Deborah took the CSA in May 2009 and sees the exam itself as being fair. The main problems with the exam were the expense and the travel. Having taken the exam, she thought it was very much as she expected. Cases were common GP problems. Four of the cases appeared regularly in revision books so she felt there were no surprises. After the exam she tells us: 'I felt that it is hard to judge how I have done because you don't really know what the examiners wanted. However, I just did what I would normally do.'

Preparing for the exam

Deborah prepared for the exam by meeting in a learning set. 'We met in a group of four from January, initially weekly, and started role playing cases. This group was formed from a larger group that met weekly in preparation for the AKT. Because we had prepared well for the AKT there was little book work in the CSA prep and we concentrated on consultations. I also went on a RCGP 2-day preparation course in Croydon, which was really useful to calm nerves on the day and ensure I knew where to stay, go, etc. It was also really useful practising cases and getting feedback from the examiners. The Deanery also organised for us to have a mock exam of four cases one Saturday with feedback. Also monthly VTS sessions have helped.'

The most helpful things to Deborah were the study group and the RCGP course.

Hannah Kundu

Hannah is 28 and also qualified in Leicester. She is engaged, and is getting married in a few months, so has spent the beginning of 2009 trying to organise the wedding and studying for exams. Following the first two foundation years, she entered a three year VTS, and has done posts in Medicine, Surgery, O&G, Urology, Neonates, A&E, Respiratory, Paediatrics and of course General Practice. She hopes to work full-time, initially in a salaried post, before becoming a partner in a few years. She would like to further develop an interest in respiratory medicine, chronic obstructive pulmonary disease (COPD), asthma and bronchiectasis management, in the primary care setting.

Reflecting on the exam

Hannah took the CSA in May 2009 and thought the exam was 'terrifying though fair' and that when used with the AKT, it was effective in assessing registrars' medical knowledge and consultation skills. Reflecting on how the exam had gone, Hannah tells us she was 'Very unsure. This seems to be a common response among my friends before the results are known. I have no idea whether I got to the nub and did OK or whether I completely missed the point, which is a bit unnerving – all will be revealed in June!'

Preparing for the exam

Hannah prepared for the exam in different ways. She did 'lots and lots of role play and joint surgeries, using the marking scheme with the positive and negative indicators to try to self-rate my normal consultations at work.' She also attended the RCGP 2-day CSA course, a deanery revision day with four patients, and the programmed day using the cases in this book. She also looked at some of the more common guidelines.

The most helpful things to Hannah were the preparation mentioned above, along with using the positive and negative markers, which really helped 'as I realised I needed to check health beliefs and understanding more and I could see the progress I was making. I think it was good doing a variety of things to try to keep the motivation going.'

Himanshu Shekhar

Himanshu is 29 and also trained in Leicester. He is happily married. He has taken a pretty typical route into General Practice, having done house jobs, a medical rotation and the VTS. He intercalated a BSc in his medical undergraduate training and his work was published. He aspires to be involved in medical teaching at all levels. 'I enjoy it and find it fulfilling. I was always starved for teaching as an undergraduate and therefore I hope to rectify it from my end at least.'

Reflecting on the exam

On the CSA, Himanshu tells us it is 'comprehensive and covers a wide variety of topics, though overly expensive'. He also asks us to note that there are 'no "real" patients and no "real" signs, which means for candidates the ability to elicit signs remains a bit of a mystery,' though he appreciates how this can be difficult for simulators to enact, given the nature of exams. He took the CSA in May 2009 and found it difficult to judge how he had done. He completed all the cases in good time, and felt he made a good attempt at addressing the different domains.

Preparing for the exam

Himanshu prepared for the CSA with a weekly learning set: 'they were awesome and really helped with practicing ideas and techniques'. He also found the group good to meet with and to talk to about issues arising in preparation and in day-to-day work. His preparation hints include:

▶ review relevant curriculum statements
▶ enact cases in groups
▶ read around topics on GPnotebook
▶ attend a couple of courses, including the local deanery one (if there is one), to get a feel for the exam.

Shamit Kalla

Shamit is 30 and trained in Bangalore, India. He is married with no children, and his past work experience includes Psychiatry and the VTS scheme, which for him also included some dermatology.

Reflecting on the exam

Shamit took the CSA exam in May 2009 and found it a challenging exam, definitely setting the bar high. However, 'unfortunately it all comes down to how you perform on the day . . . you may or may not perform up to your usual standards.'

Preparing for the exam

Shamit prepared for the exam by reading some of the published CSA books and by taking part in the simulations done as part of the ST3 programme sessions. He was also part of a learning set. His hints for exam preparation include: 'Establish your group, meet up regularly, make sure you read the theory behind the cases on your own. The more theory you know, the smoother you will appear during the CSA.'

Shiloh Jacintha Jonnalagadda

Shiloh is 32 and trained at the Christian Medical College in Vellore in India. She is married and is a mother, already juggling a career with a family, with two children aged 7 and 4. She is married to a Specialist Registrar (SpR) in Acute Medicine and Intensive Care. She worked in O&G in a Rural Mission Hospital in India, with hands-on experience in all procedures and operations, and did a medical rotation in Leicester, gaining her Membership of the Royal College of Physicians (MRCP). She then moved into General Practice and VTS training, gaining experience in Paediatrics, Psychiatry, Urology and O&G. She hopes to work as a GP using her other experience to become a GP with a Special Interest (GPwSI) in Rheumatology and Diabetes and possibly Family Planning. She is already considering becoming a trainer as well.

Reflecting on the exam

On the CSA she tells us: 'It is a valuable exam, trying to assess a GP in the different areas of communication skills and knowledge base. It is quite comprehensive but a bit elaborate. It does cover a vast curriculum.' She wonders whether it would be more objective if videoed or if there were two examiners per case like in PACES for MRCP, although she understands that this is difficult for obvious logistic reasons. She took the CSA in May 2009. She found that she couldn't quite wrap up consultations due to stress and felt it was a very artificial situation where she just couldn't be herself. The exam didn't go as well as she would have liked, and she felt quite unsure of what the cases were looking for.

Preparing for the exam

Shiloh prepared for the exam in a learning set that used case discussion and role playing. She attended one course run by the RCGP and wrote a case that is in this book. She found the most helpful preparation methods were role play and group discussion.

Mark Shaffu

Mark is 28 and is currently on the East Midlands GP Training Programme. He recently got engaged to his 'lovely fiancée Shireen' and is looking forward to the wedding this year. He supports Leicester City Football Club, which is fun but can be an emotional rollercoaster. Graduating from Leicester in 2004, he completed foundation training and went directly into a GP training programme, the e-portfolio and nMRCGP being thrust upon him. He says this was an '"interesting" transition.' His training has included a variety of specialties: A&E, Medicine, Paediatrics and O&G. He sees that his career 'has still got a long way to go, and where will I be and what will I do – dunno!! But, I do know that General Practice is what I want to do. I'm keen to follow an interest in dermatology within General Practice and develop my GP skills further.'

Reflecting on the exam

Mark sat the CSA exam in May 2009. Being in a transition group from the old style VTS to nMRCGP, this was the only sitting he was able to attempt before completion of his training, only having a six-month period in General Practice at the end of the registrar period. He says: 'The CSA exam – well, that was an experience! I was nervous, excited, panicky and relaxed all at once; an odd combination I know, but you'll know what I mean. It's an exam where experience, timing and confidence are crucial. It is very much like a regular surgery, but each patient is a demanding case. You end up leaving exhausted. It's difficult to gauge how well you've done after leaving the exam.'

Preparing for the exam

Mark found the way to prepare for the CSA included a combination of joint surgeries, reading of guidelines and theory, along with practice consultations with friends. 'With a group of other trainees, we wrote cases for each other, and used one of the CSA revision books. We carried out practice consultations under time limits and then marked each other against the CSA marking criteria. As well as practicing timing and consultation skills, it also allowed us to bounce ideas and clinical knowledge off each other.'

Vicky Taylor

Vicky is 28 and trained at Leicester University. She has lived and worked in Leicester ever since, doing her foundation and GP training there as well. In between 'Mini-Cexs, PSQs, DOPS, COTS, CBDS' she enjoys cooking and watching the Blackburn Rovers, especially if they win. She keeps the Transition Group supplied with homemade cakes. She has done a variety of different jobs including Paediatrics, O&G and Palliative Care. She sees the wide experience as having been useful in preparing for the CSA. She is interested in palliative care, and hopes to combine this with General Practice in the future.

Reflecting on the exam

Although initially terrified about the thought of Croydon's 'Tower of Terror', Vicky thought the CSA, which she took in May 2009, quite a pleasant and fair exam. She tells us that she felt 'it was a good way of assessing our consultation skills, and the cases I saw were very reflective of the type of patients and problems I see day to day. It seemed to go OK – my main problem was time keeping, and I found I hadn't quite reached the end in several cases.' Her advice would be to arrive at the exam in good time and to try to sleep well the night before. She sat in with another registrar in her practice the day before the exam, who was a great help calming her nerves.

Preparing for the exam

Vicky prepared for the exam in a learning set of five people, practising role plays with each other. They each tried to bring one or two cases to each session, picked from real life scenarios they had seen in primary care. They took turns being the doctor or patient with the rest of the group observing, timekeeping and giving feedback. She felt that this worked really well as they gave good feedback on each other's performance. It was also useful to watch other people and think about what the assessors may be looking for. She spent time reading appropriate guidelines and reading around topics using PUNS/DENS (Patients Unmet Needs/Doctor's Educational Needs).

Kafayat Lee

Kafa is 28 and trained at the University of Nottingham, graduating in 2004. Last year she got married to Adrian, who is a town planner. For fun she does a bit of Wing Chun kung fu every week. Her training has included posts in A&E, Medicine, Surgery, O&G, Paediatrics, Psychiatry and Palliative Medicine. She holds the Diploma in Child Health (DCH), Diploma of the Faculty of Family Planning (DFFP) and Diploma of the Royal College of Obstetricians and Gynaecologists (DRCOG) qualifications. She hopes to be a trainer in the future and to start a Masters in Medical Leadership in a few years.

Reflecting on the exam

Kafa took the CSA in May 2009 and thinks that for the most part it is a fair exam, although she found it difficult to judge how she had done after the exam was over.

Preparing for the exam

Kafa prepared for the exam in a study group with friends and used books and day-to-day consultations in practice as a focus for learning. She tells us: 'The study group was probably the most useful, as I got feedback from colleagues and learnt a lot from them.'

Caroline Taylor-Walker

Caroline is 29 and qualified from Southampton University. She initially went into medicine to be a surgeon and did a year of basic surgical training 'before realising that I missed the interaction with people and missed being able to help with all of their problems, so decided to go into General Practice, which was a great career move.' She has almost completed her three years of GP Vocational Training, during which time she has also done her DFFP, DRCOG and a foundation course in Acupuncture. She hopes to qualify as a GP and then do a variety of different bits before settling down in a practice. 'I have not yet decided what these variety of bits may be, but they vary from exhibition medicine to working on a cruise ship to volunteer work in Africa or even just working abroad somewhere.' She has a lot of interests including sports medicine, ENT, family planning and minor operations and is hoping that with time one of these will come through as a strong point for further pursuit.

Reflecting on the exam

She took the CSA in May 2009 and felt that it was a 'true to life' examination, testing what doctors come across on a daily basis. 'The only bad point was having to perform in front of someone with an actor patient.' She found it difficult to assess how she performed, but 'the cases were not too complicated and I felt there were no tricks. The actors were all very good and the set-up felt like a normal GP practice, which all helped the process. The hardest part is staying focused and calm in the stressful situation of the exam where you have to make decisions on the spot.'

Preparing for the exam

She prepared for the exam in a learning set of five people. 'This was a good number as most could not turn up on the same day so we always had three present. We each brought a case that we had come across in GP practice and we role played the case, each playing the patient of the case we brought along. We then gave feedback and discussed how we could improve the consultation.'

Uma Mahalingappa

Uma is 31 and trained in India. She is married to an anaesthetist, and has a daughter, Diya, who is 3. She worked in Medicine, Paediatrics and Neuro-rehabilitation in India before coming to the UK in 2003. She then did an attachment in Medicine for about four months, and worked as a FY2 in Birmingham from 2004–2005 in Infectious Diseases, Public Health and General Practice. She joined GP training in Leicester in 2006. Her aims are to have a balanced career and family life as a GP and she hopes to travel around the world if possible.

Reflecting on the exam

Uma thought the CSA, which she took in May 2009, was a good assessment of applied clinical knowledge, but perhaps not the best – the results also depending on how well the candidates can perform under stress and anxiety. As she waits for the results she is unsure how she has done.

Preparing for the exam

Uma prepared for the exam by using group discussions, role plays, videos and by attending RCGP and deanery courses. She found the most helpful aspect of preparation was the day-to-day experience with patients, videoing her consultations at work and reviewing them on her own and with her trainer.

Dave Sharma

Dave is 33 and trained at Leicester Medical School. He is single, and took a traditional course into GP training following the foundation years. He hopes to go into GP partnership, and finally settle down.

Reflecting on the exam

Dave took the CSA exam in May 2009. He tells us that 'the exam passes very quickly and is not as negative as it is made out to be.'

Preparing for the exam

Dave attended a deanery CSA preparation course and the RCGP CSA preparation course. He read the Oxford Handbook of General Practice and used the RCGP CSA DVDs, Series 1 and 2. He also did mock consultations with friends and joint consultations with his trainer. He found the most helpful things were joint consultations, practicing self-designed cases with friends and the RCGP course.

Keshdip Hayer

Kesh is 29 and graduated in 2004 from Leicester University. She was born in Birmingham, but has lived in Leicester as part of a big family since 1999. She has a passion for the fine things in life: cars, handbags, shoes . . . which helps to drive her love for shopping! She has always wanted to gear her career towards General Practice and opted for a Pre-Registration House Officer (PRHO) year, which included four months of General Practice. Following a stand-alone six-month job in Respiratory Medicine she started a traditional three-year VTS scheme, including posts in Rheumatology, Geriatrics, Paediatrics and O&G, which all proved to be of great benefit on her return to General Practice. After the Certificate of Completion of Training (CCT), she wants to locum in the Midlands to get a feel for which area she wants to settle in and what type of practice she would like to commit herself to. Eventually she would like to be a full-time partner in a practice with an interest in practice management and teaching.

Reflecting on the exam

Kesh took the CSA in May 2009 and tells us 'I personally don't feel that the fact that the exam is only held in Croydon is ideal. It is a costly exam and the travel expenses contribute to this. On the whole it is a fair exam.' On taking the exam, she felt she underestimated how quickly the 10 minutes go and the number of ethical cases there would be. She found it difficult to judge her performance after the exam and had mixed feelings about each case.

Preparing for the exam

Kesh prepared for the exam with weekly video surgeries and reflecting on these on her own and with her trainer. She did joint surgeries with her trainer using the CSA domain marking scheme. Towards the end she met up a couple of times with her peers to discuss cases. Unfortunately she was unable to do this earlier on as she was also revising for her AKT at the time and it was difficult managing revision for AKT, working life (doing evening surgeries) and revision sessions. She also used a couple of CSA revision books to aid her revision around common cases. The most helpful preparation was the video surgery, which gave her insight into ways to adapt her management plans to the patient.

Krishna Pabbaraju

Krishna is 36 and trained in India. He has been married for just over six years and has a new baby girl who keeps him and his wife busy and steady. He 'dabbled in Anaesthetics and General Medicine' and completed his VTS through placements in Paediatrics and Psychiatry.

Reflecting on the exam

Krishna took the CSA in May 2009 and thought it was a tricky examination. 'You have to do well in most stations on the day, as each case has reasonable depth and complexity. So a bad day could be expensive.' However, he felt that the cases were from traditional GP surgery, and that practice in everyday General Practice was an advantage as in the exam 'one can be in an autopilot mode without particularly striving for it'. The exam seems short: 'It finished in a blink.'

Preparing for the exam

Krishna prepared for the exam with CSA books and videos to give a baseline understanding of the format and the possible scenarios. He also found group sessions, practicing the common scenarios in small groups, particularly rewarding. The theoretical base was helped by reading the RCGP Associates in Training (AiT) newsletter and handbooks. Websites like www.patient.co.uk, www.gp notebook.co.uk, www.arc.org.uk and EMIS online resources were also very helpful. Practice sessions with friends were probably the most helpful, although assessments by the trainer in joint surgeries helped to set standards.

5

The curriculum

'And what is the use of a book,' thought Alice, 'without pictures or conversations?'

(*Alice's Adventures in Wonderland*, p. 11)

The GP curriculum

The GP curriculum is a weighty tome, although easily accessed on the web.[1] It is used by registrars on the e-portfolio. It is seen as a guide in preparing for the AKT. The curriculum consists of two main parts: the core curriculum itself, *Being a General Practitioner*,[2] and 31 interpretive statements[3] covering key subject areas. In this chapter, the curriculum is placed into context. I will demonstrate how the curriculum can be used broadly to help learning in speciality training and, more particularly, in assisting with preparation for the CSA.

The Teaching and Learning Guide

The Teaching and Learning Guide can be found on the RCGP website.[4] It seeks to describe the competences needed to be a General Practitioner, reflecting the motto of the RCGP, 'cum scientia caritas' (compassion with knowledge). In its introduction to the RCGP curriculum we are told:

> The RCGP curriculum is for UK doctors training for general practice, their trainers and educational supervisors. It covers the period known as *specialty training for general practice*: from the end of the Foundation Programme to the award of a Certificate of Completion of Training (CCT). It assumes that trainees have already attained the core competences of the Foundation Programme.
>
> Set within a framework for a structured educational programme, the RCGP curriculum identifies the knowledge, skills and professional attitudes required of a doctor intending to undertake independent practice in the contemporary UK National Health Service.
>
> Since August 2007, all UK specialty training programmes for general practice have been based on the RCGP curriculum, which has been unconditionally approved by the Postgraduate Medical Education and Training Board (PMETB). The curriculum is also the educational framework adopted by the RCGP for Continuing Professional Development (CPD) and revalidation.

The guide explores the content and context of the GP curriculum, outlining six essential domains of professional competence, which it then integrates with Good Medical Practice. The six domains are patient-focused and include:

- primary care management
- person-centred care
- specific problem-solving skills
- a comprehensive approach
- community orientation
- an holistic approach.

These domains are to be understood in the light of three essential features of General Practice, which are more doctor-focused. The first of these, *contextual aspects*, looks at the doctor in his environment, be that his work, culture or organisation. The second relates to *attitudinal aspects*, relating to the doctor's attitudes, values and ethics. The final essential feature is that of *scientific aspects* and the use of a critical and research-based approach to care, which continues and adapts in the light of new knowledge, emphasising the importance of continued learning and quality of care.

The core curriculum: Being a General Practitioner

The core curriculum is just what it says: an outline of the core curriculum for General Practice. It is required reading because it presents the six domains of competence required to be a GP in the UK. In each competence domain, specified learning outcomes are identified. The document also expands on the three essential features explained in *The Teaching and Learning Guide*, described above, defining learning aims. The core curriculum is the launching pad for the subsequent interpretive statements.

The practical exercise laid out in Box 5.1 will help you to reflect on the core curriculum, relating this to your own strengths and to the CSA.

BOX 5.1 Practical exercise in familiarisation with the core curriculum

Practical exercise

1 Read the core curriculum: *Being a General Practitioner*. What are your strong areas?

2 How could a case in the CSA assess all six domains of competence?

3 Could the essential features also be assessed? How?

The interpretive statements

The 31 interpretive statements expand on the core curriculum. They endeavour to apply the core curriculum to the variety of situations seen by the practicing GP. Each interpretive statement defines specific learning outcomes relating to the six competence domains and three essential features. The statements should be used as a dynamic guide to learning. They should not be seen as a restricted or limited unchangeable syllabus that is set in stone.

In writing the cases for this book, the team of registrars were asked to look at the relevant curriculum statement and choose two or three learning outcomes to guide their writing. It is recommended that if you do write your own cases, you use a similar model. By reading the curriculum statement in a focused way, in order to choose specific learning outcomes, you will increase your understanding of the contents of the different curriculum statements. This will almost certainly enable the identification of further learning needs and encourage the development of strategies to address them. These learning needs can then be easily transferred to the PDP on the e-portfolio.

The interpretive statements are listed below.[5]

- The General Practice Consultation
- Personal and Professional Responsibilities
  — Clinical Governance
  — Patient Safety
  — Clinical Ethics and Values-Based Practice
  — Promoting Equality and Valuing Diversity
  — Evidence-Based Practice
  — Research and Academic Activity
  — Teaching, Mentoring and Clinical Supervision
- Management
  — Management in Primary Care
  — Information Management and Technology
- Healthy People: promoting health and preventing disease
- Genetics in Primary Care
- Care of Acutely Ill People
- Care of Children and Young People
- Care of Older Adults
- Gender-specific Health Issues
  — Women's health
  — Men's health
- Sexual Health
- Care of People with Cancer and Palliative Care
- Care of People with Mental Health Problems
- Care of People with Learning Disabilities
- Clinical Management
  — Cardiovascular problems
  — Digestive problems
  — Drug and alcohol problems
  — ENT and facial problems
  — Eye problems
  — Metabolic problems
  — Neurological problems
  — Respiratory problems
  — Rheumatology and conditions of the musculoskeletal system
  — Skin problems

Practical exercise

To begin to get to grips with using and applying the core curriculum and the interpretive statements, you may find it useful to do the practical exercise given in Box 5.2. A worked example of this exercise is given in Box 5.3.

The example used for the exercise can be *any* case. It does not need to be one that could be a 'CSA case'. Reflective learning on *any* scenario will improve your clinical wisdom, which is an essential attribute in the wonderfully complex and uncertain world of the General Practice consultation. It is important not to become so CSA-focused that you miss out on other opportunities that will help you develop your core skills, knowledge and professional attitude, which will make you a better consulter. This, after all, is what the CSA is really looking to assess.

BOX 5.2 Practical exercise in applying the curriculum

Practical exercise
Identify a patient that you have seen as an emergency in the last week.
Read the curriculum statement: *Being a General Practitioner*.
- What domains are relevant to your emergency case?

- What essential features are relevant to the case?

Look through the interpretive statements:
- Which statement headings are relevant to this case?

Choose one statement and identify three relevant learning outcomes
- 1
- 2
- 3

What personal educational needs can you identify?
- Knowledge gaps

- Necessary skills

- Desirable attitudes

BOX 5.3 Worked example of the practical exercise in applying the curriculum

Practical exercise
This is not a case that could easily be assessed in the CSA. However, many generic competences are demonstrated.

The patient
A 25-year-old lady with an erythrodermic skin rash needs an urgent dermatology

opinion. She speaks limited English. Apparently the dermatology registrar has told switchboard that he is not to be bleeped.

Being a GP – relevant domains

- Domain 1 – Primary care management
  - 1.3 To coordinate care with other professionals in primary care and with other specialists.
  - 1.4 To master effective and appropriate care provision and health service utilisation (understanding the processes of referral into secondary care and other care pathways).
- Domain 2 – Person-centred care
  - 2.3 To communicate, to set priorities and to act in partnership.
- Domain 3 – Specific problem-solving skills
  - 3.2 To selectively gather and interpret information from history taking, physical examination and investigations, and apply it to an appropriate management plan in collaboration with the patient.
- Domain 4 – A comprehensive approach
  - 4.3 To manage and coordinate health promotion, prevention, cure, care, rehabilitation and palliation.
- Domain 6 – A holistic approach
  - 6.1 To use bio-psychosocial models, taking into account cultural and existential dimensions.

Being a GP – essential features

- Context
  - 2 Being aware of the impact of overall workload on the care given to the individual patient and the facilities (e.g. staff, equipment) available to deliver that care.
- Attitude
  - 3 Having an awareness of self: an understanding that their own attitudes and feelings are important determinants of how they practice.
- Scientific
  - 2 Having a thorough knowledge of: the scientific backgrounds of pathology; symptoms and diagnosis; therapy and prognosis; epidemiology; decision theory; theories about the forming of hypotheses and problem-solving; preventative healthcare.

Relevant interpretive statements

- Promoting Equality and Valuing Diversity
- Care of Acutely Ill People
- Skin Problems

Choose one statement and identify three relevant learning outcomes

- Care of Acutely Ill People
  - — Recognise and evaluate acutely ill patients.

— Decide whether urgent action is necessary, thus protecting patients with non-urgent and self-limiting problems from the potentially detrimental consequences of being over-investigated, over-treated or deprived of their liberty.
— Demonstrate an awareness of the tensions between acute and routine care and impact of workload on the care given to the individual patients.

What personal educational needs can you identify?

- Knowledge gaps: how to get an urgent dermatology review at this particular hospital.
- Desirable attitudes: to avoid judgemental irritation at an unavailable registrar.

References

1 The curriculum is available at: www.rcgp-curriculum.org.uk (accessed 10 July 2009).
2 Royal College of General Practitioners. *Being a General Practitioner*. Version 1.1, February 2009. Available at: www.rcgp-curriculum.org.uk/PDF/curr_1_Curriculum_Statement_Being_a_GP.pdf (accessed 20 November 2009).
3 The interpretive statements are each available from: www.rcgp-curriculum.org.uk/rcgp_-_gp_curriculum_documents/gp_curriculum_statements.aspx (accessed 10 July 2009).
4 Royal College of General Practitioners. *The Teaching and Learning Guide*. Version 3.2, December 2008. Available at: www.rcgp-curriculum.org.uk/pdf/curr_The_Learning_and_Teaching_Guide_dec08.pdf (accessed 3 November 2009).
5 Available at: www.rcgp-curriculum.org.uk/rcgp_-_gp_curriculum_documents/gp_curriculum_statements.aspx (accessed 10 July 2009).

6

Writing your own cases

The White Rabbit put on his spectacles. 'Where shall I begin, please your Majesty?' he asked.

'Begin at the beginning,' the King said gravely, 'and go on till you come to the end: then stop.'

(Alice's Adventures in Wonderland, p. 128)

Writing your own case is one of the best ways to get into the head of the examiner. By doing this you will work out what is being looked for, but it also will help your consultation skills more generally. The fact that you have to be specific and write things down is part of this process. You will have to ask yourself, and answer, a number of questions. What is the elbow pain *really* like? What *is* the patient concerned about and why? How do you do an examination to confirm or refute the possible diagnosis of intermittent claudication? What information will the patient give and when? What does the doctor have to do to get the information? How will the patient react to a suggested management plan?

Assessment domains

The CSA is assessed in three domains. As we have seen, the first two domains, those of Data Gathering and Clinical Management, are more of the 'white coat' skills, whereas the Interpersonal Skills domain looks more at the 'cardigan' aspects. While domains may change with time, essentially they will need to look at clinical competence and communication. The present explanations of the three domains were given in Box 2.1.

Writing a case

The easiest way to write a case is to use a template. This makes sure that there are few gaps for even the most excellent consulter to identify. If the doctor wishes to find out about the patient's job, and the impact of the problem, you will need to have decided this in the case writing, or the case may go in a very different direction to how you planned it. However, you don't need to consider how to give a 'standardised performance' where every candidate is presented with exactly the same patient and story. As you are not writing the case for a reliable high stakes exam, this rather complex and time-consuming task is not necessary. A three-part template that can be used for writing cases is given in Boxes 6.1 to 6.3 on the following pages.

BOX 6.1 Template for writing cases – Part 1

CSA case preparation document
Part 1
Name:
Age:
Sex:
Ethnicity:
BMI:
Special visual features:

Presenting problem:
What is the diagnosis or problem when framed?
Curriculum statement:

Learning outcomes from curriculum statement:
1
2
3
4

What knowledge is needed for this case?

What is the current evidence relevant to this case?

Where can the evidence be found?

BOX 6.2 Template for writing cases – Part 2

Part 2
What are you looking for:
- in history?
- on examination?
- in management?

What is needed for a good consultation?

What will an above average registrar do?

What will an average registrar do?

What will a below average registrar do?

BOX 6.3 Template for writing cases – Part 3

Part 3
What will the patient say when they come in?

Describe the presenting problem.

a. For a symptom:
- What is it?

- Where is it?

- Does it radiate?

- When did it start?

- How did it start?

- What is it like?

- How bad is it?

- What does it stop the patient doing?

- Any triggers?

- How has it developed over time?

- Any exacerbating or relieving factors?

- Any associated features?

What diagnoses might relate to this problem?

What questions would you expect the candidate to ask to rule in and out other possible diagnoses? What are the answers to these questions?

b. For a problem:
- What happened or has been happening?

- How did it all start?

- How have things developed?

- What is happening now?

- How has it affected the person?

- How has it affected others?

- Has anything helped to make things worse or better?

- Anything else that has contributed to the problem?

How might this problem be framed?

What questions would you expect the candidate to ask to try to crystallise what the key problem is and what are the answers?

Consider the patient's ideas, concerns and expectations
- What does the patient think is going on and why?

- What do particular words or concepts mean to the patient?

- Why do they think this?

- What particularly are they concerned about? Why?

- What are they wanting or expecting? Why?

Cues
- What verbal cues will the patient give?
  — How will they give them?

  — What words are key?

  — What happens if the candidate doesn't pick them up?

- What non-verbal cues will the patient give?
  — How will they give them?

  — Dress?

- — Affect?

- — Body language?

- — What happens if the candidate doesn't pick them up?

Psychosocial
- What is the home situation?

- Family and friends?

- How is the problem impacting?

- Lifestyle
  - — Drugs

  - — Smoking

  - — Alcohol

  - — Sexual behaviour

  - — Belief systems

- How does the patient spend his time?
  - — Work?

  - — Hobbies?

  - — What does he do?

  - — How is the problem impacting?

Examination
- What will be found on examination?

- How will this be demonstrated?
  - — Exam card? What will it say?

  - — Actual examination? What will it demonstrate?

Management
- What will the patient expect in management?

- What will the patient accept in management?

- How involved will they be in the management?

- What questions will they ask?

- What will they do if they are unhappy with the management?

Patient record
- Put together a patient medical record sheet
  — Blood results? Well (wo)man check? Smears? Medication? Allergies?

Stages to a good case

When writing a case to use in a learning set, the following 12 stages will help to guide you through the process.

Stage 1: choose the subject area

The first thing to do in writing a case is to choose the subject area to consider. If working in a team, make sure that the cases you each write cover the breadth of the curriculum and that you are not all doing the same subject area. Ideally, choose a curriculum statement relevant to an area in which you are less able. For example, a female doctor may identify men's health as being a weak area, and will be willing to prepare a patient story on a man with a prostate problem. In a similar way, a male doctor may use his choice of case to learn more about HRT or PMT.

For the Transition Group CSA training day, described in Chapter 4, case areas were allocated to cover a variety of aspects of the curriculum, as indicated in Table 6.1 below. This is where the complexity of life makes a difference. One registrar, Deborah, who couldn't come to the day, still wrote a case, whereas others who were planning to write cases didn't, but came along anyway. Flexibility is of the essence. Others wrote cases and were sick on the day. This will happen in learning sets too.

Stage 2: examine the curriculum statement

Examine the curriculum statement related to the case. Look at this broadly. Don't just rush to tick the boxes. Use the time to identify any learning needs that you could note down and add to your e-portfolio. Then try to think of a patient you have seen that had a problem that could be adapted to fit some of the learning outcomes. Choose the learning outcomes you are going to write the case to fit and write them down.

TABLE 6.1 Case allocations for the CSA training day

	Name	Patient	Statement	Difficulty	Emphasis
1	Deborah	Male 33	Sexual health	Moderate	Domain 3 Evidence-based element
2	Vicky	Male 6	ENT and facial problems	Easy	Domain 1 New problem Mum presents
3	Caroline	Male 55	Healthy people: promoting health and preventing disease	Moderate	Domain 2 Ongoing problem
4	Mark	Male 26	Digestive problems	Difficult	Domain 3 New problem
5	Krishna	Male 48	Cancer and palliative care	Moderate	Domain 2 Preventative element
6	Uma	Male 42	Metabolic problems	Difficult	Domain 3 Emphasis on ICE
7	Hannah	Male 66	Mental health	Easy	Domain 1 New problem
8	Shiloh	Male 47	Men's health	Moderate	Domain 2 Emphasis on bio-psychosocial
9	Kesh	Female 33	Genetics in Primary Care	Difficult	Domain 3 Possible serious diagnosis
10	Dave	Female 15	Clinical ethics and values-based practice	Easy	Domain 1 New problem
11	Kafa	Female 25	Skin problems	Moderate	Domain 2 Ongoing problem
12	Shamit	Female 35	Neurological problems	Difficult	Domain 3 Unrealistic patient expectations
13	Himanshu	Female 45	Women's health	Easy	Domain 1 Evidence-based element

Stage 3: consider the knowledge base

Think about what knowledge base is needed to address the issues the case presents. Look for the latest evidence, for example on NICE or SIGN, or if none of these cover the subject area, other national or local guidelines. Consider how the diagnosis is usually made and what the management options could be in a typical case. Really get your head around the knowledge base and add this to your learning log on the e-portfolio. It may be that you want to do something slightly different, for example a complaint. Just use the same process. For example, find out about the practice, local and national complaints policies and try to understand how they could be applied in the context of a 10-minute 'consultation'.

Stage 4: what should a GP registrar do?
Decide what it is reasonable to expect a GP registrar to do in this case and write it down. Be specific about what you are expecting in the history, examination, management and interpersonal aspects.

Stage 5: define levels of performance
Define what you think an average, a good and a poor performance would be. Be specific. Rather than say 'investigate appropriately', specify what those appropriate investigations might be and what you might expect good, average and poor registrars to do. By committing yourself on paper, your colleagues can more easily challenge you to justify what you were expecting and why, which will help your more general learning.

Stage 6: picture the patient
Picture the patient. And remember you are going to have to role play them. Consider their age, sex, appearance, BMI and any other visual features that will serve as cues. For example, an Asian gentleman of 50 years is more likely to visually cue the need for CVS screening than is a 16-year-old girl with body piercings. In the latter case, however, you may well be thinking risk-taking behaviour and chlamydia. In your learning sets, you will need to give this extra information to the doctor before the consultation starts. In the exam itself, go with the visual cues that you are given.

Stage 7: fully describe the problem
Describe the presenting problem *fully*. For example, if you are looking at a frozen shoulder you will need to describe:
 ▶ where the pain is
 ▶ where it radiates to
 ▶ what it's like
 ▶ how bad it is
 ▶ what its impact has been
 ▶ what it feels like
 ▶ how long it has been there
 ▶ how it started and has varied over time
 ▶ whether it has been there before
    — if so, when and how did it resolve
 ▶ what makes it better
 ▶ what makes it worse
 ▶ any other symptoms that are associated with it.

If it was your receptionist complaining about your practice manager, you could use a similar information-gathering approach, using open questions so that you can clarify what she has come about and what has actually happened or is happening. You could explore when it happened, what led up to it and what has happened since, identifying factors that seem to make the situation worse or better, or anything else that the receptionist has noticed that may be relevant. Using a similar process you can clarify most problems that could be presented.

Stage 8: summarise the problem

Summarise the presenting problem in your own words, and write it down.

Stage 9: what are the likely diagnoses?

With this presenting problem, consider what the diagnoses could be. List each likely one, remembering the probabilities of disease. If you walk in the British countryside in summer, you are more likely to see a horse than a giraffe. In the same way, if you are presented with a patient with a cough and a fever, a viral upper respiratory tract infection (URTI) is higher on your list than Plasmodium falciparum. If, however, the patient saw the nurse four weeks ago for travel advice before going to India and you can see that they were given malaria tablets, malaria may become one of the important diagnoses you would like to exclude.

For each reasonable diagnosis, consider what open and closed questions a doctor might ask in order to rule diagnoses in and out. Decide what the answers should be to move the doctor in the right direction. If the doctor comes out with any questions you have not identified, the answer will have to be 'no'.

Stage 10: identify ICE

Identify the patient's ideas, concerns and expectations. You will need to decide what the patient thinks is going on and why. If they say that they think they are having a heart attack, you will also need to decide what they understand a heart attack to be and what it means to them. They could just see it as a death sentence and have no idea of what the underlying pathology and aetiology are. However, you could decide your patient is a cardiac nurse who is already thinking about the advantages and disadvantages of a coronary artery bypass graft (CABG) as compared to angioplasty and who might know more about it than the doctor does. You will have to do some reading here, to improve your own knowledge in this area.

Clarifying the patient's view of words like 'arthritis', 'colitis', 'ME' or even 'bunion', will help you describe your patient's narrative. This will automatically lead in to looking at their worries and what they expect the doctor to do and why they expect them to do it. Once you have decided on this you will then need to determine what the doctor has to do to trigger them into giving this information and whether they are going to cue this verbally or non-verbally. Is the patient going to come in looking worried? Are they going to use words like 'serious' or 'concerned'? All of this needs to be defined.

Also determine the psychosocial aspects of the case, defining the home and work life of the patient and their social network. This will include necessary lifestyle issues, but make these appropriate for the case, with as few blind alleyways for the consulting doctor to go down as possible. Remember, you are aiming for a 10-minute consultation.

Stage 11: what are the likely examinations?

Consider, in the light of all the information above, what possible diagnoses could the doctor be thinking of? Remember horses not giraffes, but also remember that rare illnesses do happen. Think what examination the doctor might do to prove or disprove their hypotheses, and decide what the findings would be. You then need to decide whether you want the doctor to do an examination or not. This will probably depend on how complex the rest of the case is, as time will be an issue. If an examination can be done in the time, decide how you will give the findings. This could be by simulating abnormal findings or by giving an examination card. The card should be directed to be given after the doctor has indicated what they want to examine.

Stage 12: management plans

Think what the ideal management options would be and decide what the patient's response to each of them would be if they are given a choice of management. Decide what questions the patient would ask to clarify things, and what the patient will say if asked about their understanding of the management plan and follow-up. Consider what an appropriate follow-up would be and decide what the patient would say if asked what they want to do about follow-up.

Once you have gone through all 12 stages, read through the case again, critically tidying up the details. Then get a colleague, or even your trainer, to go through it and see if they can see any other areas that could be tidied up or developed further. Print out enough copies for your learning set. Meet up as a learning set and run the case.

7

Marking cases and giving feedback

'Speak English!' said the Eaglet. 'I don't know the meaning of half those long words, and, what's more, I don't believe you do either!'

(Alice's Adventures in Wonderland, p. 31)

One of the most important aspects of working together as a learning set is to help each other learn. Feedback is essential to make this happen and, to be effective, feedback needs to be challenging and yet supportive. Like the Heinz 57 varieties of consultation models, feedback tools also come in many varieties. The most popular method in GP teaching appears to be what has become known as Pendleton's model,[1] although many teachers of consultation skills use Agenda-Led Outcome Based Analysis (ALOBA)[2] and SET-GO,[3] which emphasise the learner's agenda, observation and goals. As the learning process described in this book focuses on the team, the method of feedback I will describe is the TEAM method.[4]

▶ T: Timing
▶ E: Environment
▶ A: Appropriateness
▶ M: Manageability

If all four factors are suitably included in providing feedback, this will facilitate learning for all those involved. We will consider each factor in turn.

Timing

In the learning sets, the best time for feedback is after an observed consultation performance. A copy of the form in Box 7.1 is filled in by each observer, as well as by the person playing the patient and by the doctor taking the consultation.

The doctor is the first to give feedback, sharing their thoughts on the consultation, emphasising both strengths and weaknesses, giving an example of each to back up their judgements. This latter feedback technique involves making a point and then illustrating it with an example of where and how that point occurred. The doctor can then suggest what he thinks could have been done differently and how this could have been done.

The observers can then give feedback on their thoughts on the observed consultation, again backing up each point with an example and giving other suggestions for improvement. Finally, the patient can give feedback on their own thoughts and perceptions.

Environment

As with all feedback, the environment needs to be appropriate. This includes using a room with privacy. Receiving challenging feedback can be more beneficial if given in a supportive group environment, but not if outsiders are listening in. This is particularly relevant as many learning sets meet in people's homes and not in a more specific learning environment. A useful point to remember is that food, such as coffee and cake, can implicitly make feedback seem more acceptable!

Appropriateness

Feedback needs to be appropriate. The level of challenge and support need to be adapted to the situation and to the person receiving the feedback. If someone is having a crisis of confidence, or the cat has just died, the element of support needs to be greater. If the exam is beckoning, and your dear colleague has missed what to you is a glaring cue, yet again, a more direct challenge, relying on the long-term supportive relationship you have built up, may be a good way forward.

The feedback needs to be specific and about an observable behaviour. It should not make judgemental interpretations on what has been observed or about what others were thinking. 'You appeared to move a lot in your seat, and I *wondered* if you were nervous' is suggestive, but is not judgemental. 'You *were* really irritated and angry' interprets observed behaviour in a judgemental way. The former encourages the learner to respond; the latter can engender defensiveness. In a similar way, just saying 'that was great' without saying *what* the doctor did that was great and *why* it was great, doesn't help to reinforce the good practice.

Manageability

Feedback needs to be manageable. One 'good' point followed by six 'bad' points is pretty disempowering. It is really important to balance the feedback and to prioritise the most important areas. On the feedback form in this chapter only two positive and two developmental areas are asked for. The formalising of the feedback in writing ensures that the two positive aspects are not overlooked, but it also allows for the learner to see repetitive themes emerging.

At the end of the feedback time, the person playing the doctor can summarise for the group the key strengths that she is taking away and the two areas that she plans to work on, specifying how she will do this. The rest of the group can then identify their own relevant individual learning needs that have come out of the process and can share these with the group as well, saying what they are going to do and how. This way the feedback results in specific, measurable, achievable, realistic and timely (SMART) learning objectives for all those involved.

BOX 7.1 Feedback form

Name of case:

Name of doctor:

Would you say the performance you observed was:

- Above average
- Average
- Below average

Why?

Do you think this performance would:

- Pass
- Fail
- Not sure

Why?

What two things did the doctor do well? How did she do these?

What two things could be done to improve the performance of the doctor in this case? How could she do this?

References

1 Pendleton D, Schofield T, Tate P, *et al. The New Consultation.* Oxford: Oxford University Press; 2003.

2 Silverman J, Draper J, Kurtz SM. The Calgary-Cambridge approach to communications skills teaching. 1: Agenda-led outcome based analysis of the consultation. *Educ Gen Prac.* 1996; 7: 288–99.

3 Silverman J, Draper J, Kurtz SM. The Calgary-Cambridge approach to communications skills teaching. 2: SET-GO method of descriptive feedback. *Educ Gen Prac.* 1996; 8: 16–23.

4 Knight R. Giving and receiving feedback. In: Hastings A, Redsell S, editors. *The Good Consultation Guide for Nurses.* Oxford: Radcliffe Publishing; 2006. pp. 115–6.

8

CSA case example 1

'And how many hours a day did you do lessons?' said Alice, in a hurry to change the subject.

'Ten hours the first day,' said the Mock Turtle: 'nine the next, and so on.'

'What a curious plan!' exclaimed Alice.

'That's the reason they're called lessons,' the Gryphon remarked: 'because they lessen from day to day.'

(Alice's Adventures in Wonderland, pp. 103–4)

The case below can be used as an example of how to write a case. It is not perfect, so look for the loopholes that could be tidied up. You could also use this as a practice case if some of the learning set have not read it. It emphasises the importance of patient-centred consulting skills, as well as an up-to-date understanding of pre-conceptual issues. The taking of herbal medicine, the need for travel vaccines and the unrealistic patient expectation add unpredictable, but true to real life, complexity.

Janine Jamieson: pre-conception care
Part 1

Name: Janine Jamieson
Age: 36
Sex: Female
Ethnicity: Any
BMI: Normal
Special visual features: Smart, well turned out lady, wearing jeans and a T-shirt

Presenting problem: Pre-conception care
What is the diagnosis or problem when framed: Advice relating to planning a pregnancy
Curriculum statement: Women's health

Learning outcomes from curriculum statement:
1 Recognise that many women consult for lifestyle advice, and that GPs should not over-medicalise these issues.
2 Demonstrate an understanding of the importance of risk factors in the diagnosis and management of women's problems.
3 Outline prevention strategies relevant to women (e.g. safer sex, pre-pregnancy counselling, antenatal care, immunisation, osteoporosis).

4 Understand the importance of promoting health and a healthy lifestyle in women, and in particular the impact of this on the unborn child, growing children and the family.

What knowledge is needed for this case?
▶ Pre-conception healthcare advice.

What is the current evidence relevant to this case?
▶ Self-care.
▶ Alcohol.
▶ Body weight.
▶ Folic acid.
▶ Fish.
▶ Vitamin A.
▶ Vaccinations and screening tests.
▶ Immunisations.
▶ Cervical screening.
▶ Advice for men.

Where can the evidence be found?
www.nhs.uk/Conditions/Preconception/Pages/Recommendations.aspx?url=Pages/what-is-it.aspx

Part 2
What are you looking for?
A doctor who can take a good history from the patient, identify why she has come, identify what she wants to get out of the consultation and give the necessary information to the patient in an understandable way.

What is needed for a good consultation?
▶ A focused, patient-centred history.
▶ Identification of the patient's ideas, concerns and expectations.
▶ Appropriate advice given to the patient in a patient-centred way.

What will an above average registrar do?
An above average registrar will:
▶ Take a fluent, focused, organised patient-centred history
  — menstrual history
  — sexual history
  — past and present gynaecological history
▶ Quickly pick up and explore the patient's cues, identifying the patient's thoughts, feelings and concerns about a possible pregnancy
▶ Address these concerns giving appropriate information and advice in a patient-centred way
▶ Give advice on diet, alcohol, folic acid, exercise, rubella vaccines, diet and holiday vaccines/medication in pregnancy
▶ Give advice to avoid herbal medicines
▶ May include advice for the partner, e.g. smoking and alcohol.

The above average registrar will pick up on the patient's unrealistic expectations and try to reframe them:

- 30% will conceive within one month
- 60% in 6 months
- 85% in a year.

What will an average registrar do?

An average registrar will take a reasonable history from the patient, identifying the patient's relevant past and present gynaecological history in a reasonably organised way. They will explore the patient's cues, identifying the patient's thoughts, feelings and concerns about a possible pregnancy. They will address most of these concerns giving adequate information and advice in a patient-centred way.

What will a below average registrar do?

A below average registrar will take a poor, unfocused history from the patient. They will fail to identify much of the patient's relevant past and present gynaecological history and the history will be disorganised. They will fail to pick up or explore the patient's cues, or to identify the patient's thoughts, feelings and concerns about a possible pregnancy. They will fail to address concerns, giving inadequate information that is not tailored to the patient. They will ignore the risk of travel vaccines, malaria protection and pregnancy. They will not recommend folic acid, stopping herbal medication or decreasing alcohol intake. They may be very doctor-centred.

Part 3

What will the patient say when they come in?
'Hello. I have come to talk about having a baby.'

Describe the presenting problem

- Wanting to get pregnant.
- Currently on the pill.
- Wanting a child at the end.
- Planning a last baby-free holiday to India in 4 months.
- Never been pregnant before.
- Works as a lawyer.
- Not done much reading so far.
- Periods started age 13.
- Went on pill at 20.

How might this problem be framed?

- Wanting pre-conception advice.

What questions would you expect the candidate to ask to try to crystallise what the key problem is and what are the answers?

- Non-smoker.
- Drinks 2 large glasses of wine most days.
- Gets little exercise.
- Diet: eats when she has to – chocolate, coffee, wine and fruit.
- Little protein and vegetables.

- But poor diet is OK as she takes herbal medication from the local Chinese herbalist – not too sure what it is . . . just to keep her healthy.
- No FH of abnormality.
- Husband is also a lawyer.
- A baby 9 months after the holiday would be perfect.
- Smears up to date.
- 1 of 3 children herself and no FH of fertility problems.
- SI 2–3 times a week.
- No STD in the past.
- 2 previous partners.
- Both she and her husband went to the GU clinic before they started having sex.
- Check up clear.
- Husband not been married before and is not a father.
- Going to Kerala in South India for a 2-week holiday in 3 months.

Consider the patient's ideas, concerns and expectations
- Wants advice.
- When should she come off the pill?
- Is there anything else she should do?
- Thinks getting pregnant is easy and is not expecting any delays or problems.
- Expecting to get pregnant the month she stops contraception.
- Thinks she might stop pill (Microgynon) before she goes on holiday.
- Knows she needs travel vaccines and anti-malarials but has not thought about this and pregnancy.
- Does not know what travel vaccines she needs.
- No reading on pre-conception care, which is why she is here.

Cues
What verbal cues will the patient give?
'I know I will get pregnant easily . . .'
'I don't want to get pregnant before the holiday . . .'
'The herbal medicines will keep me healthy . . .'

What happens if the candidate doesn't pick them up?
They will be turned into questions in the management time.

What non-verbal cues will the patient give?
Confident and in control.
Used to life going her way.

Psychosocial
- Married for 5 years, to a lawyer husband.
- He works in company law.
- She is a family lawyer.
- High powered work – long hours, good income.
- In control of life.
- Parents live in Manchester, siblings in Canada and Edinburgh.
- Both younger, both professionals and neither married.

- Have a group of friends from work but relationships are rather superficial.
- Enjoys good holidays.
- Not much time for socialising.
- Likes opera and theatre.

Examination
None required.

Management
What will the patient expect in management?
- Advice given in an evidence-based way.

What will the patient accept in management?
- Advice backed with a degree of evidence, e.g. avoiding herbal remedies, as not sure what is in them and may harm baby; need to take folic acid to decrease chances of abnormalities like spina bifida.

How involved will she be in the management?
- Will be very interactive in management – asking why to suggestions.
- Happy to take these on board.
- If doctor indicates she may take a while to conceive, she will show shock but take the information on board.

What questions will she ask?
- When should I stop the pill then?
- Cue questions if not picked up.

What will she do if she is unhappy with the management?
- Will show that she is unconvinced and will ask where she can find out more.

Patient record
Janine Jamieson
36 years old
8 The Archway

PMH
Nil of note
Smears UTD
BP 116/70 taken 2-months ago

Medication
Microgynon

SH
Non-smoker

Running this case

The case is run as described in Chapter 3 under the sub-heading 'Meet as a group and run a mini-surgery' of Step 7. One of the group, who knows the case to be run, plays Janine. One member of the group who does not know the case is given a copy of the Medical Record and plays the doctor. The rest of the group read the case notes and the descriptions of the level of registrar performance, observe the consultation, and fill in the feedback form given in Box 7.1. Verbal feedback is given in a supportive way, the case is discussed, learning points and learning needs identified, and actions for the next session defined and allocated. Written feedback forms are then given to the consulting doctor.

At the end of the process, each doctor can fill in a reflection sheet to formalise their learning, which can then be attached as evidence for the e-portfolio. This is the bit that is often rushed over, but for those of you who are more reflective in learning, it may be worth returning to this at a later stage, in order to consolidate and direct your further study. A template for producing a reflective account can be found in Box 8.1.

BOX 8.1 Template for a reflective account of a CSA training case

Reflective account
Name of case:
Your name:
Curriculum statement:

I watched/discussed/wrote/consulted with this case (please circle)

What did I learn from writing this case?

What did I learn from discussing this case?

What did I learn from watching this case?

What did I learn from consulting with this case?

9

CSA case example 2

'I think I should understand that better,' Alice said very politely, 'if I had it written down: but I'm afraid I can't quite follow it as you say it.'

(*Alice's Adventures in Wonderland*, pp. 96–7)

Twenty per cent of GP consultations involve seeing a patient with a skin problem. In this case, the patient has a changing skin lesion and is concerned about what it could be. As in many consultations, the patient's understanding has been affected by her experience and in order to address her concerns the doctor needs to explore and take on board her health understanding. Two very useful resources for skin problems are listed in the evidence section.

The case uses the same template as CSA case example 1, but is written in a more narrative form. Personally I prefer the narrative form, as it helps me imagine and 'act' the patient more easily. Try to write cases using each method and consider the differences you identify.

Kim Jarman: changing mole
Part 1
Name: Kim Jarman
Age: 32
Sex: Female
Ethnicity: Caucasian
BMI: Normal
Special visual features: Skin not badly sun damaged

Presenting problem: Concern about a mole
What is the diagnosis or problem when framed? A nurse concerned about a changing mole
Curriculum statement: Skin Problems

Learning outcomes from curriculum statement:
1 Make timely appropriate referrals on behalf of patients to specialist services, especially to rapid-access pigmented lesion (sometimes called skin cancer, mole or melanoma) clinics.
2 Identify the patient's health beliefs regarding skin problems and either reinforce, modify or challenge these beliefs as appropriate.
3 Recognise the risk of inappropriate referrals and under referrals.

4   Ensure that skin problems are not dismissed as trivial or unimportant by healthcare professionals.

What knowledge is needed for this case?
▶ Diagnosis and management of pigmented skin lesions.
▶ Risk factors of melanoma.

What is the current evidence relevant to this case?
Atypical naevi:
▶ can be larger than typical naevi
▶ have variable colour and shape
▶ are usually found on the trunk, buttocks and scalp
▶ are more common on sun-exposed areas
▶ are more common in those with fair skin and freckles
▶ have an increased risk of developing a melanoma
▶ do not all need to be removed
▶ can be monitored using photographs
▶ should be protected from sun
▶ should be referred to a dermatologist if:
  — they change in size, shape or colour
  — they are causing diagnostic uncertainty.

Where can the evidence be found?
http://dermnetnz.org/lesions/atypical-naevi.html
www.pcds.org.uk/image-atlas/a-z-of-diagnosis/50-image-atlas-detailed-articles/
    113-atypical--dysplastic-melanocytic-naevus

Part 2
What are you looking for?
A registrar who can take an appropriate history of a changing skin lesion, identify the patient's health beliefs, reach a shared understanding of the problem, relating this to the patient's concerns and refer appropriately to secondary care.

What is needed for a good consultation?
▶ A focused history.
▶ Appropriate choice of examination and interpretation of findings.
▶ A negotiated management plan that addresses the patient's concerns.

What will an above average registrar do?
An above average registrar will clarify the reason the patient has come, identifying what has precipitated presentation now. They will pick up and explore both verbal and non-verbal cues leading to a greater understanding of the patient's concerns. They will gather relevant information on the patient's history of a changing skin lesion and on relevant risk factors in a patient-centred way, recognising a possibly serious condition and explaining to the patient what they think is going on and why, referring appropriately to rapid access pigmented lesion clinic or equivalent. They will address the patient's inaccurate health beliefs relating to melanoma. They may give sun

advice and will safety net appropriately. They will support the patient in coping with uncertainty, and will not falsely reassure.

What will an average registrar do?
An average registrar will clarify the reason the patient has come, gathering relevant information on the patient's history of a changing skin lesion. They will identify that the patient has a possibly changing atypical mole, recognising the presentation of a potentially serious condition. They will refer to the rapid access pigmented lesion clinic or equivalent, safety netting appropriately. They will identify some of the patient's ICE and will address some of these.

What will a below average registrar do?
A below average registrar will fail to define the nature of the problem or to take a focused history of a patient with a changing skin lesion. They will fail to explore risk factors for malignancy or to identify that the patient has a changing atypical mole, and may not recognise the presentation of a potentially serious condition. They may refer inappropriately, e.g. through choose and book. They will fail to pick up cues relating to the patient's ICE and occupation, and will not address the patient's inaccurate beliefs about melanoma prognosis. May be falsely reassuring, overly bleak in prognosis or show little understanding or concern.

Part 3
What will the patient say when they come in?
'Hello. I am quite worried. I have a mole that seems to be changing.'

Describe the presenting problem
▶ Has had this mole on her thigh, since she was a teenager she thinks, but over the last year she thinks it might have been getting a bit bigger and darker.
▶ It is on the side of her upper thigh on the right and is about one cm across.
▶ She thinks that it was smaller in size last year and thinks it was less dark, but she is not sure.

What diagnoses might relate to this problem?
▶ Benign naevus.
▶ Atypical naevus.
▶ Malignant melanoma.
▶ Seborrhoeic keratosis.
▶ Dermatofibroma.

What questions would you expect the candidate to ask to try to crystallise what the key problem is and what are the answers?
Only give this information if the doctor asks specifically.
▶ It has not crusted and it is not itchy.
▶ Pigment is a bit irregular you think, but it has always been that way, but seems to have got bigger.
▶ No other symptoms at all.
▶ You do not use a sunbed and hate sunbathing as you burn easily.
▶ You are of celtic origin (Scottish).

- You have no other moles that you are worried about.
- You have about 4 others on your trunk.
- They have not changed at all.
- You have never lived abroad.
- There is no FH of cancer of any kind.
- You have not injured yourself and cannot remember ever having had an insect bite there.

Consider the patient's ideas, concerns and expectations

- If the doctor asks about your concerns:
  - Indicate that you are concerned it might be a melanoma (use the word melanoma as this is a cue that you may be medical). You think a melanoma is a nasty form of skin cancer that spreads and kills you in all cases. You don't think people survive melanomas and you don't think there is any form of treatment for this. You have not had many people in the hospice with melanomas though and you haven't done much reading on it at all.
- If the doctor explores your initially volunteered concern or tries to find out why you are here now:
  - Indicate that you had a patient who was very similar to you in the hospice recently who died of a melanoma, which has made you more concerned. You have coped with the patient's death and don't need to explore this further as the hospice has good support mechanisms. However, as you are worried you think your mole should be removed and checked. You think it needs to be cut out and looked at under the microscope.
- If the doctor picks up from your notes that you work in the local hospice and explores this:
  - Indicate that you think this is why you are concerned. If doctor explores this further, give more of your concerns as above.

Cues
Friendly, open, good eye contact, but mildly anxious.
Use technical words like melanoma to cue nursing background.

Psychosocial
You are a nurse at the local hospice and enjoy your work very much. You trained as a general nurse and then when a part-time post came up at the local hospice you moved over as it fitted with the children. It works well. You haven't done much extra training apart from the ongoing training at the hospice. You are married to Ed, who is an estate agent manager. He is with a local company and his job is stable. You have two children: Sam aged 10 and Susie aged 8. They are fit and well and at the local school. Your parents live in Scotland and are fit and well. You are Scottish too but have lost your accent. You keep fit and well and go jogging 3 or 4 times a week with a friend. You are a non-smoker and very, very rarely drink alcohol. Your husband had a vasectomy 4 years ago. No more children are planned.

Examination
If an examination is requested you will ask what the doctor wants to look for and why. You will then give a copy of the examination card below.

> **Examination card**
>
> *Kim Jarman*
>
> Generally freckled skin, but no marked sun damage
>
> 4 normal looking moles on trunk
>
> 1 cm naevus on thigh
>
> No lymphadenopathy
>
> The concerning mole on the thigh is 1 cm in diameter, with irregular pigment. The central area is very dark. You think it is an atypical naevus. You do not think this is a melanoma, but are not completely sure.

Management

You are pretty sure you need to be referred, but if the doctor explains that he thinks it is nothing serious and explains what he thinks it is and what needs to happen, you will be relieved and very happy to accept his advice.

If the doctor indicates that he thinks it is a definite melanoma you will go quiet and say that you thought it might be. If you are given the opportunity, you will share your concerns if you have not done this already. If you have been given the opportunity to share your concerns earlier, you will not want to talk about it any more but will want to go away and think about things and wait for the hospital appointment.

If the doctor indicates that he is not sure but that it needs to be checked urgently by a specialist you will be happy with this and your anxiety level will drop a little knowing you are being taken seriously. You will then want to know what they might do and how quickly it will be done in an information-gathering way rather than a panic/anxiety way.

If given the opportunity and not already explained, you will want to know:
- Do you think it is a melanoma?
- Melanomas can never be cured, can they?
- Will you refer me?
- What will they do?
- How soon will they see me?
- If offered an appointment more than a week away ask:
  — Can't I be seen sooner?
  — What do I do if I don't hear anything?

Patient record

Kim Jarman
32 years old
6 Coles Close

PMH
Nil of note
Smears UTD
BP 110/70 taken 6 months ago

Medication
Nil

SH/FH
Non-smoker
Less than 1 unit of alcohol per week
Exercises 3–4 times a week
Nurse at local hospice

Running this case

The case is run as in the previous chapter. The only difference is that here there is an examination card to be handed over by one of the observers. It is worth checking out what everyone thinks is required for examination in the CSA, referring back to Chapter 1 if necessary. The process is then started:

1 one of the group plays Kim
2 one member of the group is given a copy of the Medical Record and plays the doctor
3 the rest of the group read the case notes and descriptions of the above average, average and below average doctor
4 observe the consultation and fill in the feedback form
5 verbal feedback is given in a supportive way
6 the case is discussed
7 learning points and learning needs are identified
8 actions for the next session are defined and allocated
9 written feedback forms are given to the consulting doctor
10 reflection sheets are completed and added to e-portfolio.

Practice CSA cases

Robert Davies by Deborah Webb

Consultation with a gentleman who has testicular pain
Part 1
Name: Robert Davies
Age: 33
Sex: Male
Ethnicity: White/any
BMI: Normal
Special visual features: Casually dressed, jeans, well kempt, appears anxious/embarrassed about presenting to the doctor

Presenting problem: Testicular pain
What is the diagnosis or problem when framed? Epididymo-orchitis – importance of taking a sexual history
Curriculum statement: Sexual Health

Learning outcomes from curriculum statement:
1 Manage primary contact with patients who have sexual health concerns and problems.
2 To recognise the causes of acute testicular pain.
3 Take a sexual history from a patient in a way that is private and confidential, non-judgemental, responsive to the reactions of the patient and avoids assumptions about sexual orientation or the gender of the partner(s), assumptions related to age, disability or ethnic origin.
4 Recognise availability of GUM clinics as a referral option.

What knowledge is needed for this case?
Be able to recognise and distinguish the important causes of acute testicular pain:
▶ strangulated hernia
▶ torsion of the testis
▶ torsion of the hydatid of Morgagni
▶ acute epididymo-orchitis
▶ haematocoele
▶ appendicitis
▶ tumour.

Be able to take a sexual history:
- when did you last have sex?
- casual or regular partner?
- how many partners?
- did you use condoms?
- how long have you been with him/her?
- male and/or female partners?
- accurate description of sexual practices including:
  — anal sex – insertive/receptive/both
  — oral sex – insertive/receptive.

STDs or other symptoms in partner:
- discharge
- dysuria
- itching
- rashes
- sores
- lumps.

What is the current evidence relevant to this case?
- In patients you suspect may be at risk of STI, it is important to send urine for chlamydia/MSU.
- Patients should be offered a referral to GUM (in this case it would be refused).
- If you suspect STI then in under-35s ceftriaxone 250 mg IM stat + doxycyline 100 mg BD 10/7 (difficult in non-GUM setting).
- In over-35s, ciprofloxacin 500 mg BD 10/7 to cover enteric organisms (in this case this would be reasonable as he is low risk for STI).

Where can the evidence be found?
www.bashh.org/documents/31/31.pdf

Part 2
What are you looking for?
The candidate should in a sensitive and non-judgemental way be able to put the patient at ease in order to exclude important causes of testicular pain.

What is needed for a good consultation?
- A focused history.
- The need for examination put in a sensitive way.
- Negotiation with the patient with regard to management: epididymo-orchitis should strictly speaking be referred to GUM but this patient wants you, his doctor, to treat him.
- Investigation – urine dipstick and MSU/chlamydia.

What will an above average registrar do?
An above average registrar will take a fluent, focused patient-centred history, whilst putting the patient at ease. They will quickly pick up his cues about being embarrassed and be able to easily explore his sexual health. They will understand his feelings that he

wants to be treated by the doctor today. They will exclude serious causes of symptoms, for example testicular torsion. They will be able to provide appropriate advice in regard to sexual health if questioned, e.g. if they bring up the possibility of chlamydia, they will be able to inform the patient about this. Appropriate treatment and advice given, with good safety netting.

What will an average registrar do?
An average registrar will take a reasonable history from the patient. They will explore the patient's cues, identifying the patient's thoughts, feelings and concerns about a possible STI. They will address most of these concerns, giving adequate information and advice in a patient-centred way. Appropriate treatment and advice given.

What will a below average registrar do?
A below average registrar will be insensitive to the patient's embarrassment about the problem.

They will miss out the sexual history part and focus on surgical causes. They will be unable to provide appropriate advice and management. They will be doctor-centred and will not take on board the wishes of the patient to be treated in primary care.

Part 3
What will the patient say when they come in?
Patient will sit down and look to the floor. On prompting he will say 'I have a pain'.

Describe the presenting problem
- He has had the pain for nearly a week.
- It gradually came on one day.
- It is in his left testicle.
- There has been no trauma.
- The pain is usually there and can be quite severe at times, but there are no aggravating or relieving factors that he can identify.
- It hasn't stopped him doing anything.
- His pain does not radiate anywhere.
- He has come as the pain is persisting, getting slightly worse and he is worried about cancer.
- He has had some mild dysuria a week ago but this is not a prominent symptom.
- No vomiting, bowels normal.
- No fever.
- He is in a long-term relationship of 2 years.
- Female partner, long-term, vaginal and oral intercourse only.
- He denies any other recent partners.
- He has no urethral discharge, itching, rash, sores or lumps.
- He had chlamydia 3 years ago and was treated at the time.
- Partner well.
- No anal sex, no other sexual relationships in last 2 years.

Consider the patient's ideas, concerns and expectations
- The patient is worried that he has cancer.
- The word 'chlamydia' to him means STI and therefore unfaithfulness.

▶ He wouldn't go to GUM if suggested because he wants treatment today and does not have time.
▶ Has a fully booked schedule and cannot take time off easily.

Cues
What verbal cues will the patient give?
If prompted he will say he is worried about cancer, although he doesn't know anything about testicular cancer.

What non-verbal cues will the patient give?
Will look to the floor to show embarrassment.
Difficulty maintaining eye contact initially.
If the doctor is empathetic the patient will become more at ease.

What happens if the candidate doesn't pick them up?
He will continue to look worried and will indicate verbally that he is worried, but will not say he was worried about cancer, unless explicitly asked what his worries are.

Psychosocial
▶ Is a self employed plumber, good work life, not stressed but is busy.
▶ Partner of 2 years, Jo-Anne.
▶ No problems.
▶ Currently living together.
▶ Plays football and keeps fit.
▶ Couple of pints at weekends and non-smoker.

Examination
Will be happy to be examined, but will ask what is being looked for. Examination card can then be given.

> ### Examination card
> *Robert Davies*
> Left-sided tenderness of the testis, with some scrotal erythema and oedema
> Palpable swelling of the epididymis
> Testis normal in position
> No urethral discharge
> No nodes
> Apyrexial and looks well
> Pulse 68 BPM and BP 120/80
> Does *not* look like a testicular torsion

Management
▶ The patient will want an explanation of what the doctor thinks is going on.
▶ The patient will accept antibiotics and investigations but will ask what antibiotics? How should he take them? What will they do?

▌ The patient will understand when explained the need to rule out STI. But will ask if this means his partner has been unfaithful.
▌ The patient will not be happy if the doctor does not manage him and suggests that he seeks help from GUM.
▌ The patient will be happy if the doctor indicates that he needs to look up or find out what he should give.

Patient record
Robert Davies
33 years old
72 Stirling Way

PMH
Eczema as a child
Nil else; rarely attends doctor

Medication
Nil

SH
Lives with girlfriend.
Non-smoker, moderate drinker.
No drug use.

11

John Bradford by Hannah Kundu

Consultation with a gentleman who is tired all the time (TATT)
Part 1
Name: John Bradford
Age: 66
Sex: Male
Ethnicity: Any
BMI: Normal
Special visual features: Casually but appropriately dressed in clean jeans and jumper

Presenting problem: TATT
What is the diagnosis or problem when framed? Depression
Curriculum statement: Care of People with Mental Health Problems

Learning outcomes from curriculum statement:
1 Describe the need to check for psychological illness whilst avoiding the habit of checking extensively for physical illness: ideas about the physical, psychological and social should be integrated in both consultation and investigation of illness.
2 Suicide risk assessment.
3 Manage people experiencing mental health problems in primary care, bearing in mind that several interventions may be effective for each mental health condition, including different forms of talking therapy, medication and self-help.
4 Demonstrate how to screen, and diagnose, people experiencing mental health problems, using effective and reliable instruments where they are available.

What knowledge is needed for this case?
The candidate must be:
▶ able to assess a patient for symptoms of depression
▶ able to risk assess a patient for suicide risk in a sensitive manner
▶ aware of how moderate depression is managed.

What is the current evidence relevant to this case?
▶ Mild depression – 'watchful waiting', CBT, counselling, exercise.
▶ Moderate depression – consider an SSRI as first line along with the above.

- In moderate depression to continue antidepressant for 6/12 after symptoms have remitted before reducing (2 years if recurrent/relapsing).
- PHQ9 validated for use in primary care.
- DSM IV/ICD10 criteria.
- SSRI – as effective as a tricyclic but with fewer side effects, therefore to be used first line.

Where can the evidence be found?
www.nice.org.uk/guidance/CG90
www.patient.co.uk/health/Depression.htm
www.library.nhs.uk/mentalhealth
www.bap.org.uk/pdfs/antidepressant.pdf
www.nhs.uk/conditions/Depression/Pages/Introduction.aspx?url=Pages/What-is-it.
  aspx

Part 2
What are you looking for?
- Initially an open consultation, focusing down to ask specific questions to complete the history, identifying patient's ideas, concerns and expectations, exploration of the patient's health beliefs and understanding and a patient-centred approach.

What is needed for a good consultation?
- Good systematic history, excluding quickly the physical causes for TATT and concentrating on depression as a cause.
- Open/sensitive questions allowing patient to 'open up'.
- Risk assessment in a sensitive manner.
- Exploration of the patient's understanding and health beliefs.
- Exploration of the patient's ideas, concerns and expectations.
- A negotiated shared management plan.
- An exploration of the possibility of combining medication and CBT/counselling and lifestyle advice.
- Appropriate follow-up and safety netting.

What will an above average registrar do?
- Quickly rule out a physical cause for TATT.
- Allow sensitive exploration of patient's feelings in an open manner.
- Show empathy.
- Ask about the patient's understanding of depression and his health beliefs.
- Explore the patient's ideas, concerns and expectations.
- Discuss with the patient the management options and form a shared management plan, looking at different options, combining medical and lifestyle advice.
- Ensure appropriate follow-up and safety netting.
- Patient-centred approach.

What will an average registrar do?
- As above, appropriate history and management plan, but may not explore patient's understanding and health beliefs as well as an above average candidate.
- May do all the above but with less empathy and connection with the patient.

What will a below average registrar do?

- Unsystematic history, areas of relevant history missed, failure to pick up on cues.
- Failure to assess suicide risk, or assessment made but in an insensitive manner.
- Patient's ICE, understanding and health beliefs not explored.
- Doctor-centred.
- Lots of closed questions, not allowing patient to explore his feelings.
- Management plan given to patient, rather than shared.
- Management plan not in accordance with generally accepted views on the appropriate management of depression.

Part 3

What will the patient say when they come in?
'I am sorry to trouble you but my wife has asked me to come to see you.'

Describe the presenting problem

- Wife says that she is fed up with him always complaining that he is tired.
- Symptoms all gradually occurred over the last 6 months since he retired. Now they are getting worse.
- Beginning to feel that he needs help, unsure what to do or why he feels like this. Therefore doesn't know if anything can be done to help him.
- Mr Bradford is finding it difficult to get to sleep. When he gets to sleep he finds that he wakes a lot. Once awake after 4 am he is unable to get back to sleep.
- If the candidate explores sleep issues sensitively – 3 daughters now at university – youngest daughter left home 6 months ago.
  — Mr Bradford used to wait up for them to get home at night.
  — Now they are not there still seems to be waking.
- No known symptoms of any medical condition – no DM/thyroid symptoms or red flags regarding a tiredness that could be related to a cancer diagnosis etc.
- Mr Bradford's wife is worried that he is always complaining that he feels tired.
  — She asked him to come to the doctors.
  — She is unable to come with her husband as she is playing tennis with her friends.
- If explored sensitively – patient retired 6 months ago from busy accountant job, did well at work, worked hard and felt that he was well respected and useful.
- Wife has never worked; she has a good social network of female friends with whom she meets up regularly. He feels that he is now useless with no purpose and often left at home whilst she goes out.
- No other relationship difficulties, but feels things have changed a bit since he retired. His life has changed but hers has continued the same.
- Patient loves his wife, knows that she loves him. They have always had a good relationship.
- If asked – does admit to feeling low, doesn't see how things can improve.
- Does enjoy meeting up with his old colleagues every now and again or if he goes out with wife.
- Mr Bradford is worried because he has lost his temper a few times when his children have asked for more money – not violent but he has shouted at them. This is unusual for him as he is usually laid-back.
- Concentration reduced.
  — Unable to concentrate on the crosswords he usually likes to do.

- Anxiety – not a problem, 'never suffered with me nerves'.
- Appetite – lack of interest but does eat well.
  - Good balanced diet as his wife is a good cook.
  - No weight loss.
- Risk assessment – no suicidal ideation.
  - Mr Bradford has his family to think of, wants to see his children graduate.
- Finances – OK. Worked hard to raise enough money to put his children through university and to provide for his retirement with his wife. He is proud that he has managed to achieve this.
- Sexual relationship with wife – 'not as much as when we were younger but no problems in that department'.

What diagnoses might relate to this problem?
- Moderate depression.
- Physical causes can be quickly excluded.

What questions would you expect the candidate to ask to rule in and out other possible diagnoses?
- Explore problems with sleep.
- Ask about symptoms associated with physical conditions that can make patients tired/low.
- Find out about his low mood.
- Explore the changes in his life that have occurred over the last 6 months and how these have impacted on his self-esteem and self-worth.
- Ask about any suicidal ideation.
- Ask about family history.
- Explore social history.
- Discuss with patient his ideas about why he is feeling like this.
- Explore patient's understanding of depression.
- How would the patient like his depression to be managed?

Consider the patient's ideas, concerns and expectations
Ideas – Mr Bradford is unsure why he is unable to sleep. If the candidate explores with him the idea that he appears quite low/depressed he is open to this suggestion. Mr Bradford feels that he may have known deep down that he is depressed but didn't want to admit that it could happen to him. Mr Bradford agrees, if depression is explained well to him, that he probably is depressed.

Concerns – Mr Bradford's brother has had depression over the last 20 years. His brother has said in the past that he has been unable to come off his antidepressants without relapsing. Mr Bradford is concerned about this:
- does this mean he is addicted to his medication?
- will he become addicted?
- will he be on antidepressants all his life?

His brother has never tried to harm himself and does manage to continue working whilst depressed.

Expectations – Mr Bradford would like his symptoms to be treated and for him to be well again.

- He is amenable to any management plan if well explained, although he does not feel that he needs counselling.
- Mr Bradford is open to starting an SSRI if it is explained to him (how long he will need to take it, that he will not be addicted to them but will need to slowly reduce to avoid withdrawal symptoms).
- He is very reluctant to accept an SSRI if this is not explained.
- Mr Bradford does not feel that he needs counselling at the present.
- He is open to talking to his wife about how he feels, trying to do more activities with her and looking at trying to increase his exercise by playing tennis.
- He would also be interested in part-time voluntary work as he feels that this might help him feel more worthwhile.

Cues
What verbal cues will the patient give?
'My problems all started 6 months ago after I retired.'
'My children are all at university.'
'My wife could not come with me today because she is playing tennis with her friends.'
'When I was working, I felt useful, respected. I was providing for my family.'
If cues regarding the changes in his life are not noticed, he will not offer the information about how he now feels about himself or his feelings of low mood.

What non-verbal cues will the patient give?
Mr Bradford speaks at a normal rate but his tone changes. He speaks positively with good eye contact when you discuss his life pre-retirement but when talking about his feelings and his life at present, he appears more negative and with reduced eye contact.

What happens if the candidate doesn't pick them up?
Mr Bradford will again not be as likely to give the candidate information about his low mood and feelings of low self-worth.

Psychosocial
- FH: brother has depression.
- DH: nil.
- Married for 25 years. Wife is a patient at the practice, treated for blood pressure but otherwise is very well.
- Exercise – if asked – occasional walks, would like to do more. He is interested in playing tennis with his wife or friends.
- Never smoked.
- Alcohol – 'a few pints of beer at the weekend'.

Examination
None needed. If the registrar asks to carry out an examination, the patient should ask what they want to do and why. One of the observers will then state to the registrar that the examination result is normal.

Management

▶ The patient will want a good explanation of depression.

▶ If starting an SSRI he would like information about how to take it, side effects, how long he will need to take it. He will also want to be reassured that he will not become addicted to his antidepressant.

▶ He expects to be involved in deciding how his condition should be managed.
  — Once it is explained that he is depressed, he will not accept watchful waiting as he has been feeling low for over 6 months.
  — He will accept an SSRI if all above is explained.
  — He will not accept counselling as he does not feel he has any issues to discuss.
  — He will accept the idea of talking to his wife and increasing what they do together.
  — He will also accept the idea of some voluntary work if offered – he thinks that this might make him feel useful again.
  — He is happy to think about increasing the amount of exercise he does, especially if this is done in a social context, e.g. playing tennis with friends.

▶ Mr Bradford will ask questions about the treatment plan and generally be quite positive about trying to 'help himself'.
  — If involved he will be a well-motivated patient.

▶ Mr Bradford will not be happy if the management plan is given in a doctor-centred way where he is not allowed to feel involved in his treatment.
  — If the approach is doctor-centred he will become uninterested and not engage with the plan.

▶ Mr Bradford will not be happy if only offered watchful waiting or counselling.

▶ If this occurs he will become frustrated and state that 'this isn't going to help me', 'how can I go on feeling so awful', 'I don't need counselling'.

▶ If an SSRI or lifestyle advice are not offered he will ask if he can talk to another doctor.

Patient record

John Bradford
66 years old
33 Causeway

PMH
Appendicectomy aged 21 years

Medication
Nil

SH
Non-smoker
10 units of alcohol per week
BP 120/80 and bloods at well man check a month ago
IHD risk low
No FH IHD

12

Eva Peterson by Shamit Kalla

Consultation with a 35-year-old lady with headaches
Part 1
Name: Eva Peterson
Age: 35
Sex: Female
Ethnicity: Any
BMI: Low BMI
Special visual features: Smartly dressed wearing a business suit, talks on a mobile phone as she enters your consultation room

Presenting problem: Headaches
What is the diagnosis or problem when framed: Migraine
Curriculum statement: Neurological problems

Learning outcomes from curriculum statement:
1 Manage primary contact with patients who have a neurological problem.
2 Recognise that neurological conditions often affect patients during their working lives, and consequently have a large impact on the family's social and economic well-being.
3 Important causes of headache – raised intracranial pressure, thunderclap headache (subarachnoid haemorrhage, enlarging aneurism or migraine), temporal arteritis, trigeminal neuralgia, herpes zoster, cancers.

What knowledge is needed for this case?
The registrar needs to be able to deal with a demanding patient with unrealistic expectations, taking a history to diagnose migraine, while excluding symptoms and signs of serious disease. They then need to manage appropriately.

What is the current evidence relevant to this case?
▶ The evidence for this can be found in a useful summary of SIGN guidance in a 2008 BMJ article.[1]

Triggers for migraine
▶ food (tyramine, alcohol)
▶ weather
▶ visual/auditory factors (bright lights, loud noises)
▶ sleep (excessive or lack of)

▶ emotional factors (stress, anxiety)
▶ hormonal (menstruation, menopause, OCP)

Treatments (BASH guidelines, see link below)
▶ Step one: over-the-counter analgesic ± anti-emetic
▶ Step two: rectal analgesic ± anti-emetic
▶ Step three: specific anti-migraine drugs
▶ Step four: combinations

Where can the evidence be found?
http://216.25.88.43/upload/NS_BASH/BASH_guidelines_2007.pdf
www.patient.co.uk/DisplayConcepts.asp?f=1&maxresults=&WordId=migraines
http://familydoctor.org/online/famdocen/home/tools/symptom/502.html
www.bmj.com/cgi/content/full/337/nov20_1/a2329?ijkey=TPs6QosisH0tqqF&keytype
=ref
www.who.int/mediacentre/factsheets/fs277/en/

Part 2

What are you looking for?
A registrar who can deal with a patient demanding a referral, take a focused history diagnosing migraine, identifying why the patient has come and what she wants to get out of the consultation. The registrar also needs to manage the problem appropriately, giving the necessary information to the patient in an understandable way.

What is needed for a good consultation?
▶ Skill for dealing with a patient demanding a referral.
▶ A focused, patient-centred history.
▶ Identification of the patient's ideas, concerns and expectations.
▶ Appropriate advice given to the patient in a patient-centred way.
▶ Reassurance and provision of information and evidence to justify your thoughts on management.

What will an above average registrar do?
An above average registrar will let the patient vent their frustration initially before focusing in on the patient's expectations (i.e. neurology referral). They will then uncover the patient's health beliefs and the effect of her symptoms on her personal and professional life, exploring family history and ruling out relevant red flags. The decision to refer or not is not important. However, the above average candidate will provide further information on what migraines are and options for treatment, e.g. avoiding triggers and treatment of acute attacks. The candidate should demonstrate a logical, empathetic approach.

What will an average registrar do?
An average registrar will take a reasonable history from the patient, identifying various symptoms and excluding serious disease in a reasonably organised way. They will explore the patient's cues, identifying the patient's thoughts, feelings and concerns. They will address most of these concerns, giving adequate information and advice in a patient-centred way. They will deal with the initial frustration reasonably.

What will a below average registrar do?

A below average registrar will take a poor, unfocused history from the patient. They will fail to exclude possible red flags and not be able to elicit a psychosocial history. The history will be disorganised. They will fail to pick up or explore the patient's cues, or to identify the patient's thoughts, feelings and concerns. They will fail to address concerns, giving inadequate information that is not tailored to the patient. They may be very doctor-centred and so escalate the patient's frustration.

Part 3

What will the patient say when they come in?

'Hello, I've had these awful headaches and I need to see a neurologist.' (Said in a brusque, irritated and frustrated way.)

Describe the presenting problem

- Headache started 3 days ago, 2 separate episodes lasting 12 hours each. Now not present. Left-sided. Throbbing.
- Initially flashing lights and some tingling/paraesthesia left side of face and left arm.
- Had a similar episode 6 months ago.
- Wants a referral.
- No prior management.
- Cannot take time off work.
- Works as an investment banker.
  — 'credit crunch' – bankers under lots of pressure.
- Single, no children, successful.
- Has a sister-in-law who is a neurologist in the US.
- Grandmother had migraines.
- Took paracetamol and ibuprofen, but didn't really help.
- Not currently in a sexual relationship.
- No contraception.
- Went to optician 2 days ago for check up and all was OK.
- Nurse did her BP yesterday . . . was 110/70.

How might this problem be framed?

Patient wants a referral to neurology for her severe headaches.

What diagnoses might relate to this problem?

Migraine

What questions would you expect the candidate to ask to try to crystallise what the key problem is and what are the answers?

- Smoker – 10 cigarettes per day.
- Drinks 2 large glasses of wine most days.
- Gets little exercise due to long hours at work.
- Diet: eats when she has to – plenty of coffee, eats out frequently, take-aways.
- No contraception.
- A bit more stress than usual.
- If exam is offered will accept but will ask what the doctor wants to examine and why.

Consider the patient's ideas, concerns and expectations
▶ Expects a referral.
▶ Wants management strategies.
▶ Thinks she may have some form of serious headache, as the ones she has had have been so debilitating.
▶ Thinks migraine is a mild headache and an excuse people use for time off work.
▶ Thinks everyone (in the US) with headaches gets scans and is seen by a specialist.
▶ Has had conversations with sister-in-law who has suggested that she must see a neurologist (without knowing the mechanics of the NHS).

Cues
Comes in the room very frustrated. Has been waiting half an hour to be seen. She has not got time to waste.

What verbal cues will the patient give?
'My sister said I needed to see a specialist . . .'
'I cannot underperform at work . . .'
'I'm sure it's serious . . .'

What happens if the candidate doesn't pick them up?
They will be turned into questions in the management time.

What non-verbal cues will the patient give?
Confident and in control.
Knows what she wants, strict and firm.
Wants things done immediately.

Psychosocial
▶ Work is stressful, works long hours, hard times in the banking sector.
▶ Is an investment banker with a large bank in the city, which has received bad press lately.
▶ The headaches are taking their toll on the patient and she cannot miss work as her job is under threat in the current climate.
▶ Single and happy with this.

Examination
If the registrar wishes to examine the patient, she will ask what the doctor wants to examine and why. After a suitable response, the observer will then give the examination card below to the registrar.

Examination card
Eva Peterson
BP 120/80
Fundoscopy normal
Neurological exam normal

Management

What will the patient expect in management?

▶ Referral to neurology (as discussed with sister-in-law). If this is offered immediately, then she will ask what to do for future headaches.

What will the patient accept in management?

▶ Ideally a referral, but after some negotiating, will accept general advice, evidence in the form of leaflets and a reasonable management plan that will prevent/manage her headaches so she can work efficiently.

How involved will they be in the management?

▶ Will be very interactive in management – asking 'why' to suggestions.
▶ Reasonably happy to take these on board with some persistence.
▶ If doctor does not seem to listen and declines neurology referral, will become more difficult and demanding.
▶ Challenging.

What questions will she ask?

▶ What will get rid of them?
▶ How do you know there's nothing wrong with my brain?
▶ Cue questions if not picked up.

What will she do if she is unhappy with the management?

▶ Will continue to insist on an urgent neurology opinion, and if she feels she is not getting anywhere will give up and decide to go privately.

Patient record
Eva Peterson
35 years old

PMH
Smear UTD and normal
BP 110/70 yesterday (done on practice calibrated machine in the waiting room)
No pregnancies
No other relevant PMH

Medication
Nil

Reference

1 www.bmj.com/cgi/content/full/337/nov20_1/a2329?ijkey=TPs6QosisH0tqqF&key type=ref (accessed 25 May 2009).

13

Jane Doe by Himanshu Shekhar

Consultation with a 45-year-old lady with sweating

Part 1

Name: Jane Doe
Age: 45
Sex: Female
Ethnicity: Caucasian
BMI: about 25
Special visual features: Smartly dressed lady with a suit on

Presenting problem: Menopausal symptoms
What is the diagnosis or problem when framed? Giving advice relating to the meno-pause
Curriculum statement: Women's health

Learning outcomes from curriculum statement:
1 Recognise that many women consult for lifestyle advice, and that GPs should not over-medicalise these issues.
2 Demonstrate an understanding of the importance of risk factors in the diagnosis and management of women's problems.
3 Outline prevention strategies relevant to women.
4 Understand the importance of promoting health and a healthy lifestyle in women.

What knowledge is needed for this case?
Healthcare advice relating to menopause.

What is the current evidence relevant to this case?
▶ HRT – its benefits and risks.
▶ Other agents – SSRIs, clonidine, herbal remedies.

Where can the evidence be found?
www.patient.co.uk/showdoc/27000591
http://cks.library.nhs.uk/menopause/evidence/references
www.ouls.ox.ac.uk/__data/assets/pdf_file/0004/17266/Menopause_and_HRT.pdf
www.gpnotebook.co.uk/simplepage.cfm?ID=1288699910

Part 2

What are you looking for?

A doctor who can take a good history from the patient, identifying the likely diagnosis of peri-menopause while excluding other possible causes, for example thyroid disease. They will explore the history, looking for contra-indications and relative contra-indications to HRT treatment. Having identified the patient's ICE, they will explain treatment options in an evidence-based and understandable way, taking on board the patient's thoughts and views.

What is needed for a good consultation?

- A focused patient-centred history, making an appropriate differential diagnosis.
- Appropriate investigation, e.g. TFT and possibly FBC/CRP.
- Identification of the patient's ideas, concerns and expectations.
- Appropriate evidence-based advice given to the patient in a patient-centred way.

What will an above average registrar do?

An above average registrar will take a fluent, focused, patient-centred history from the patient, identifying the patient's relevant past and present gynaecological history in an organised way. They will consider and try to exclude other possible diagnoses. They will quickly pick up and explore the patient's cues, identifying the patient's thoughts, feelings and concerns about HRT and the menopause. They will address these concerns giving appropriate information and advice in a patient-centred way.

What will an average registrar do?

An average registrar will take a reasonable history from the patient, identifying the patient's relevant past and present gynaecological history in a reasonably organised way, and will consider other possible diagnoses. They will explore the patient's cues, identifying the patient's thoughts, feelings and concerns about menopause and HRT. They will address most of these concerns giving adequate information and advice in a patient-centred way. They may be uncertain and need to look up information on risks and benefits of the various treatments.

What will a below average registrar do?

A below average registrar will take a poor, unfocused history from the patient. They will fail to identify much of the patient's relevant past and present gynaecological history and will fail to consider other possible diagnoses. They will not pick up or explore the patient's cues, nor will they identify the patient's thoughts, feelings and concerns about the menopause and HRT. They will fail to address the patient's concerns, giving inadequate or wrong information that is not tailored to the patient.

Part 3

What will the patient say when they come in?

'Oh I really do hope that you can help me. I really can't bear the "heat", doctor.'

Describe the presenting problem

- Getting hot flushes.
- 2 months history, getting worse.
- Several times a day.

▶ Just gets hot all over and sweats. Looks red.
▶ Worse before her period she thinks.
▶ Disturbing daily life and sleep.
▶ Works as a Project Manager, non-smoker, does yoga.
▶ Has done some research on the internet and knows that there are natural and herbal remedies.
▶ Not tried anything so far.
▶ Wanted advice first.
▶ Menstrual history – menses since 13 with regular 28/3 cycles. Last 3 cycles irregular 2–4/52 with 3–7/7 bleeding.
▶ No FH or PMH of gynaecological problems.
▶ 2 pregnancies, normal deliveries, 20 and 22 years ago.

What diagnoses might relate to this problem?
▶ Menopause.
▶ Hyperthyroidism.
▶ Lymphoma.

What questions would you expect the candidate to ask to rule in and out other possible diagnoses? What are the answers to these questions?
▶ Thyroid symptoms – weight loss, increased appetite, palpitations.
▶ Lymphoma – night sweats, pyrexia, weight loss.
▶ Patient has none of these symptoms.
▶ Weight OK and otherwise well.
▶ Mum had an early menopause at 44.
▶ No personal or family history of arterial/venous thromboembolism risk or malignancy.
▶ Good diet.
▶ Non-smoker.
▶ Minimal alcohol.
▶ Not tried anything so far.

How might this problem be framed?
Wanting advice regarding the menopause and associated symptoms.

Consider the patient's ideas, concerns and expectations
▶ Thinks she is menopausal.
▶ Wants advice today and will go away and think about it.
▶ Uncertain as to when she should take treatment for menopausal symptoms or if there is there anything else she should do.
▶ Thinks herbal remedies may be beneficial.
▶ Thinks HRT has too many risks.
▶ Is concerned about osteoporosis.
    — Has read about it and knows it can be an issue.
    — Thinks it means bones get more fragile and can break.

Cues
What verbal cues will the patient give?
'I am not too sure about HRT, but think it might help prevent osteoporosis.'
'I know there is a risk of blood clots and cancer with HRT.'
'I think herbal medicines might help with my symptoms.'

What happens if the candidate doesn't pick them up?
They will be turned into questions in the management time.

What non-verbal cues will the patient give?
Confident and in control.
Used to life going her way.

Psychosocial
▶ Non-smoker.
▶ ½ bottle wine at weekends.
▶ Married, and partner has had a vasectomy.
▶ 2 grown up children at university.
▶ Works in local building society full time.
▶ No major stresses.
▶ Goes to the gym 3 times per week and swims once per week.

Examination
If the registrar wishes to examine the patient, she will ask what the doctor wants to examine and why. After a suitable response, the observer will then give the examination card below to the registrar.

> **Examination Card**
> *Jane Doe*
> BP 130/84

Management
What will the patient expect in management?
▶ Advice given in an evidence-based way.

What will the patient accept in management?
▶ Advice backed with a degree of evidence: lifestyle, SSRI, HRT, clonidine, alternative therapies.
▶ Will be happy to have blood tests.
▶ Will initially be sceptical with regards to efficacy of SSRIs in managing hot flushes and thinks they are for depression and that she is not being taken seriously.
▶ Will not want clonidine.
▶ Will be unsure about HRT and any other suggestions.
▶ Will want to go away and think about it all before deciding.
▶ She will not accept any medication that day but will want to go and think about it and come back.

Concerning possible management with herbal remedies:

> This guidance regarding alternative and complementary therapies is in response to the increased use of these strategies by women who believe them to be safer and more 'natural'. The choice is confusing. Evidence from randomised trials that alternative and complementary therapies improve menopausal symptoms or have the same benefits as hormone replacement therapy (HRT) is poor. A major concern is interaction with other treatments, with potentially fatal consequences. Some preparations may contain estrogenic compounds, and this is a concern for women with hormone-dependent diseases, such as breast cancer. Concern also exists about the quality control of production.
>
> British Menopause Society[1]

How involved will she be in the management?
- Will be very interactive in management – asking 'why' to suggestions.
- Will explore benefits and risks and will be happy to take doctor's advice on board.

What questions will she ask?
- Do you think it is the menopause?
- Could it be anything else?
- Do I need any tests?
- Cue questions if not picked up.
- What treatments are available?
- How good are they?
- What are the side effects?
- What if these treatments don't work?

What will she do if she is unhappy with the management?
Will show that she is unconvinced and will ask where she can find out more.

Patient record
Jane Doe
45 years old
48 Springfield Lane

PMH
Contraception: husband had a vasectomy
Smears all normal
2 normal deliveries, 22 and 20 years ago
Last seen 2 years ago for a chest infection

Medication
Nil

SH
Non-smoker

Reference

1   British Menopause Society. *BMS Consensus Statements: summary and practice points. Alternative and Complementary Therapies.* 5 June 2007. Available at www.thebms.org.uk/statementpreview.php?id=2 (accessed 28 May 2009). Also available at www.patient.co.uk/showdoc/27000591 (accessed 28 May 2009).

14

Melissa Smith by Dave Sharma

Consultation with a 15-year-old girl requesting contraception
Part 1
Name: Melissa Smith
Age: 15
Sex: Female
Ethnicity: Caucasian
BMI: Normal
Special visual features: Casually dressed

Presenting problem: Request for contraception
What is the diagnosis or problem when framed? Contraception request by a 15-year-old Gillick-competent individual
Curriculum statement: Clinical Ethics and Values-Based Practice

Learning outcomes from curriculum statement:
1   Skills to achieve meaningful consent by a patient to a plan of management by seeing the patient as a unique person in a unique context.
2   Ability to apply the ethical guidance on consent and confidentiality to the particular context of primary care.
3   Ability to draw on frameworks of moral reasoning to think through the issues and resolve conflicts of values.
4   Understanding that respect for patient autonomy is in essence a holistic approach. To enable a patient to make choices about how he or she wishes to live his or her life, a GP must explore what is important to the patient overall and not restrict information-sharing to clinical data.

What knowledge is needed and what is the current evidence relevant to this case?
▶ Contraception – types, effectiveness, side-effects, contra-indications.
▶ Sexual health advice.
▶ Child protection policy.
▶ Fraser guidelines/Gillick competence.

Where can the evidence be found?
www.gpnotebook.com

Oxford Handbook of General Practice
www.ffprhc.org.uk
www.nice.org.uk/guidance/PH3
www.gmc-uk.org/guidance/ethical_guidance/children_guidance/index.asp

Part 2

What are you looking for?

A registrar who identifies the reasons why the patient has come and, after assessing competence and ensuring patient safety, manages and prescribes appropriately.

What is needed for a good consultation?

- Clarification of presenting problem.
- Assessment of competence.
- Exploration of risk factors including general sexual health and pill.
- Managing and prescribing appropriately, including consideration of other methods of contraception including long-term contraception.
- Encouragement of parental involvement without breaking confidentiality.
- Facilitating patient choice in developing a shared management plan.

What will an above average registrar do?

An above average registrar will take an organised, focused history, in a sensitive and patient-centred way. They will ascertain that the patient is Gillick-competent, but unwilling to talk to her parents. Having ascertained the absence of child protection issues and risk factors for the combined pill, they will explain the different options available. They will respond to the patient's request for the pill and will explain how it is to be used in an understandable way, facilitating concordance. They will raise relevant issues, e.g. long-term contraception, failure rates, risks of STDs, missed pills, and condom use and will encourage the patient to ask her partner to have a check-up. They will ensure appropriate follow-up.

What will an average registrar do?

An average registrar will take a reasonable history, assessing competence and excluding child protection issues. They will assess suitability for the oral contraceptive pill, although they may not introduce the possibility of other possible methods, for example LARC in the form of Implanon. They will give advice on how to take the pill and minimise the chance of pregnancy. They will briefly look at the prevention of STDs. Follow-up will be appropriate.

What will a below average registrar do?

May be very doctor-centred, failing to identify the patient's wishes, or may adopt a consumerist approach and give the patient what she wants without an adequate exploration of the context. They may fail to exclude child protection issues or assess competence or risk factors for the contraceptive pills. Blood pressure exam may be omitted or done badly. May insist on parental involvement. May give the pill without the information required to ensure that the chances of pregnancy are minimised. May not address the possibility of STD, or the possibility of long-acting contraception. May decide to break confidentiality.

Part 3

What will the patient say when they come in?
'I want to go on the Pill.'

Describe the presenting problem
- Wants to have a more intimate relationship with her boyfriend, Sean, and does not want to get pregnant.
- Not had sex yet but has been talking about it with Sean. She wants to be ready just in case.

How might this problem be framed?
Under age request for contraception.

What questions would you expect the candidate to ask to try to crystallise what the key problem is and what are the answers?
- Sean is a 15-year-old classmate.
- Melissa knows it's not legal but has been told by friends that the doctor will not tell parents.
- Will probably have sex at his house when parents are at work.
- Does not want to tell her parents as it's none of their business, and they won't understand anyway.
- Been going out for a year; she is a virgin; he has had one partner – a one-off at a party when he was drunk.
- No migraine, periods started at 13, 28/3 cycles – regular as clockwork.
- Is sure mum has had no clotting problems at all. Sister (19) is on the pill and has had no problems.
- Is a non-smoker.
- Is at local school doing GCSEs – planning to go to university to study Chemistry.

Consider the patient's ideas, concerns and expectations
- Wants the pill as she knows it is very good at stopping pregnancy. Not sure exactly how to take it . . . thinks it is for 21 days then she stops. Thinks it almost always stops pregnancy unless she doesn't take it properly. Thinks the pill stops her making eggs. Learned this in biology.
- Wants to go on the pill as this is the safest method out.
- Has never heard of long-acting contraceptives and may be willing to consider these. Knows about condoms but doesn't think she will need them as she is a virgin and he has only had one partner. She doesn't like the idea of condoms anyway as they are unnatural.
- Thinks that she is not at risk from STDs because of her sexual history.
- She is quite happy to have sex and sees this as a natural progression of their relationship.
- She has not thought long term about pregnancy plans etc. She is too young to think of this.

Cues
Comes over as a confident, intelligent girl who knows what she wants. However, she is slightly worried as to how this consultation will go. She is worried that she might

be refused or that the doctor will tell her parents although she knows intellectually it is supposed to be confidential. This anxiety will increase if she thinks the doctor will tell her parents or if it looks like her contraception will be refused.

Examination
Happy to have her blood pressure taken and this can be taken by the doctor.
If asked her weight, indicate an acceptable weight for the role player's height.

Management
Patient will want to feel involved in deciding which form of contraception is best for her, and will engage in discussion. Patient wants to try OCP only, but will consider LARC. Patient will be happy to be tested for Chlamydia, but has not had sex yet so doesn't see why it is needed. She would be happy to ask her boyfriend to get a check up before they have sex.

What questions will she ask?
- The pill is the best contraceptive for me, isn't it?
- The pill is safe, isn't it?
- You won't tell my parents, will you?
- The patient will look more worried and push this if the doctor looks like he will tell parents.
- If offered a long-acting contraceptive, will ask what it is and how it is given. Will not be keen on an implant ('that sounds painful') or depot ('I hate needles'), or IUD/IUS ('I don't want anything inside me'). Again she will become more concerned.
- She wants to go on the pill, but may be willing to look at other methods if she can be persuaded that they are safer.

What will she do if she is unhappy with the management?
'What other options do I have?'
'Do I really need to be tested for STDs?'

Patient record
Melissa Smith
15 years old
7 The Grove

PMH
Vaccines up-to-date
Eczema as a child
Nil else relevant in history

Bradley Dillon by Shiloh Jacintha Jonnalagadda

Consultation with a 47-year-old gentleman with haematospermia
Part 1

Name: Bradley Dillon
Age: 47
Sex: Male
Ethnicity: Any
BMI: about 28
Special visual features: Well-educated and well-dressed, reserved

Presenting problem: An episode of blood in semen after masturbation. Lower abdominal discomfort.
What is the diagnosis or problem when framed? Idiopathic haematospermia
Curriculum statement: Men's Health

Learning outcomes from curriculum statement:

1 Demonstrate knowledge and describe the management of the key medical conditions that affect men.
2 Describe the indications for a PSA blood test, and explain its role in the diagnosis and management of prostate cancer.
3 Identify the patient's health beliefs regarding illness and lifestyle, and either reinforce, modify or challenge these beliefs as appropriate.

What knowledge is needed for this case?
Common causes of haematospermia.

What is the current evidence relevant to this case?
▶ Haematospermia is a common condition that is usually idiopathic and quite often unnoticed.
▶ Major illnesses to be ruled out are: prostate cancer, prostatitis, bleeding disorders, tuberculosis, urethral pathology.

Where can the evidence be found?
http://emedicine.medscape.com/article/457632-overview

Part 2

What are you looking for?

The registrar should be able to take an appropriate targeted history, exploring ICE and assessing how the problem is affecting him more generally. They should be able to develop a shared management plan, giving the patient the necessary evidence-based information, managing areas of uncertainty appropriately.

What is needed for a good consultation?

▶ Exploration of sensitive matters related to sexual health.
▶ Exploration of ICE and impact on psychosocial life.
▶ Negotiated evidence-based management.
▶ Appropriate management of uncertainty.

What will an above average registrar do?

▶ Will take a fluent, targeted history, ruling out relevant red flags.
▶ Will explore ICE in a fluent but patient-centred manner.
▶ Will make the patient feel comfortable, by maintaining a non-judgemental approach.
▶ Will sensitively explore the impact on the patient's psychosocial life.
▶ Will give the information on PSA screening in an understandable way, enabling an informed shared management plan, in an area of uncertainty.

What will an average registrar do?

▶ Will take a reasonable focused history, ruling out serious causes.
▶ Will explore ICE and the effect on psychosocial aspects in a less fluent way.
▶ Will give appropriate information, and make a good attempt at giving information in an understandable way.
▶ Will not be doctor-centred.
▶ Will not convey certainty in areas of uncertainty.

What will a below average registrar do?

▶ Will fail to take a structured history and rule out relevant red flags.
▶ Will fail to show sensitivity while exploring sexual history.
▶ Will make a poor attempt at exploring ICE or the psychosocial aspects of the problem.
▶ May try to hide uncertainty.
▶ Gives wrong information regarding PSA.

Part 3

What will the patient say when they come in?

'I am a bit scared. I have had some bleeding.'

Describe the presenting problem

▶ One episode of blood in semen last week.
▶ 5 days ago.
▶ Noticed blood in semen post-masturbation.
▶ Small flecks of bright red blood.
▶ Only once.

- Not too bad.
- Settled on its own and never recurred.
- No triggers.
- No h/o trauma.
- No rashes, no discharge, no urinary symptoms, no previous episodes, no problems with prostate, no temperature, no constipation, no previous STIs.

What diagnoses might relate to this problem?

- Prostatitis.
- Prostate CA.
- Urethral strictures or cysts or urethritis (STI).
- Trauma.
- Bleeding disorders.

What questions would you expect the candidate to ask to rule in and out other possible diagnoses? What are the answers to these questions?

- No other partners.
- LSI 2/7 ago.
- No anal sex.
- No sex toys.
- No dyspareunia.

Consider the patient's ideas, concerns and expectations

- He is worried – wife is worried as her father had prostate cancer needing radio-therapy, detected aged 60.
- Worried about having sex in case it recurs.
- Concerned he might need an operation, radiotherapy and or chemotherapy for prostate cancer as this is what his father-in-law had.
- Worries this might mean terminal illness.
- Thinks he needs a blood test to rule out cancer.

Cues

What verbal cues will the patient give?
'I'm worried this might mean something sinister.'

What words are key?
'sinister', 'scared to death'.

What happens if the candidate doesn't pick them up?
Will volunteer to say 'My father-in-law has been diagnosed to have prostate cancer. Could it be that?'

What non-verbal cues will the patient give?
Will be guarded and uneasy. Will relax once he can talk about his concerns.

Psychosocial

- Married for 25 years.
- Two children aged 15 and 12.
- Estate agent.

- Non-smoker.
- Two bottles of wine per week.

Examination
If an examination is requested will ask what they want to examine and why. Will then give the examination card.

> **Examination Card**
> *Bradley Dillon*
> Genital exam normal
> Abdominal exam normal
> Rectal examination normal

Management
- Is hoping to be told what is going on.
- Understands well, and wants to be involved.
- Will accept blood test, even if disadvantages explained well.
- If he is unhappy with the management, he will ask for a second opinion and ask to see the specialist.

What questions will they ask?
- Could this be just one of those things?
- What might be causing it?
- What else could it be?
- Do I need any blood tests?
- How accurate are they?
- What do you think I should do?
- What will happen if the blood test is high?

Patient record
Bradley Dillon
47 years old
9 Butterfield Drive

PMH
No PMH of note
Well man check 6 months ago CVD risk low
BP 110/70
Non-smoker

16

Frank Spencer by Mark Shaffu

Consultation with a 26-year-old man with abdominal pain

Part 1

Name: Frank Spencer
Age: 26
Sex: Male
Ethnicity: White British
BMI: Normal
Special Visual Features: Well-dressed, wearing T-shirt and jeans

Presenting problem: Heartburn pains
Diagnosis: Alcoholic gastritis
Curriculum statement: Digestive Problems and Drug and Alcohol Problems

Learning outcomes from curriculum statement:

1 Demonstrate a structured, logical approach to the diagnosis of abdominal pain.
2 Demonstrate understanding of the impact that social circumstances can have on drug misuse and that recovery is contingent on the effective management of those social circumstances.
3 Demonstrate an awareness that the causes of drug misuse are multifactorial.
4 Advise patients appropriately regarding lifestyle interventions that have an impact on gastrointestinal health, such as advice on diet and on stress reduction.

What is the current evidence relevant to this case?

▶ Identify symptoms.
▶ Red flags for relevant serious illness ruled out.
▶ Alcohol.
▶ Self-care.
▶ Other addictive tendencies, e.g. smoking, drugs.
▶ Diet.
▶ Social network.
▶ Occupation.
▶ Family situation.

Where can the evidence be found?

www.sign.ac.uk/pdf/sign74.pdf
www.cks.nhs.uk/alcohol_problem_drinking#-255011
www.dh.gov.uk/en/Publichealth/Healthimprovement/Alcoholmisuse/DH_072581

http://guidance.nice.org.uk/CG/Wave17/1
www.patient.co.uk/showdoc/40025275/

Part 2

What are you looking for?

A registrar who can take a focused history in a gentleman who has upper abdominal pain, who drinks excessively and who has had some recent domestic stresses. The registrar will raise awareness of the risks of alcohol, and will negotiate a shared management plan.

What is needed for a good consultation?

- A focused, patient-centred history.
- Exploration of the patient's health understanding of alcohol and its risks.
- Exploration of the patient's ideas, concerns and expectations.
- Sensitive probing of the psychosocial problems in this case, respecting the patient's wishes not to talk about these.
- Negotiated management plan.
- Addressing of the risks and safety issues of alcohol.

What will an above average registrar do?

An above average registrar will take a fluent, patient-centred history, ruling out important red flag symptoms. They will explore the patient's health understanding, identifying the fact that the patient has recently been drinking excessively. They will explore cues, and respect the patient's wish not to explore the social stresses he has been under. They will demonstrate the use of a screening tool for excessive alcohol drinking, e.g. CAGE. They will address the problems and give the correct information and advice to the patient in a collaborative manner, negotiating an appropriate management plan. They will probably suggest bloods tests, e.g. FBC, LFT, GGT and amylase. They will approach the consultation in a patient-centred non-judgemental manner, but will sensitively raise the risks of driving and alcohol.

What will an average registrar do?

An average registrar will take a reasonable history, identifying the relevant facts in an organised way, ruling out serious causes. They will explore the patient's ideas, concerns and expectations and health understanding. They will ascertain the extent of the alcohol problem, although they may not use a formal tool to assess this. They will develop a shared appropriate management plan, demonstrating patient-centred consulting.

What will a below average registrar do?

A below average registrar will take a poor, unfocused history, failing to rule out the red flag symptoms and failing to demonstrate and explore the excess alcohol issue. They will not demonstrate empathy, pick up on the patient's cues or elicit the patient's ideas, concerns and expectations. They will fail to address the issues demonstrated, and will not reach a negotiated management plan. They will fail to convey risks in an understandable way and will manage the problem in a doctor-centred manner.

Part 3

What will the patient say when they come in?

'Hello, I'm really having trouble with heartburn at the moment.'

Describe the presenting problem

▶ Recently getting worsening dyspepsia over past few months.
▶ Epigastric pain.
▶ Several times a week, no specific time.
▶ Lasts an hour or 2 sometimes longer.
▶ Burning pain.
▶ Does not radiate.
▶ Worse after drinking alcohol.
▶ No relieving factors.
▶ Has tried Rennies but not much good.
▶ Never had before.
▶ Not noted anything else when he gets this.

What diagnoses might relate to this problem?

▶ DU.
▶ Gastritis.
▶ Reflux disease.
▶ Pancreatitis.
▶ Malignancy unlikely.

What questions would you expect the candidate to ask to rule in and out other possible diagnoses? What are the answers to these questions?

▶ No pain elsewhere.
▶ Does not radiate to back.
▶ No weight loss.
▶ No melaena or haematemesis.
▶ Stools and urine normal colour.
▶ No hunger pain.
▶ No change in bowels or history of jaundice.
▶ Drinks 70–84 units alcohol per week, binge drinking on weekends.
  — Mainly bitter.
  — 8–12 pints Fridays and Saturdays (2.3 units per pint).
  — 2–4 pints most other nights.
  — Doesn't drive afterwards, only at 7.00am the next morning.
▶ Has never felt he should cut down.
▶ Mum does nag him a bit and says he is spending too much money on alcohol.
▶ Doesn't feel guilty about it or need a steadier in the morning.
▶ Does get a hangover at the weekends, and sometimes during the week.
▶ Doesn't get into fights.
▶ Eats reasonably as he sees his mum most evenings before he goes to pub and she cooks for him.

Consider patient's ideas, concerns and expectations

- Patient thinks this is heartburn and that it may be caused by the stress of his wife leaving, which he does not want to talk about today.
- He hasn't really thought about alcohol being a trigger and he thinks all this fuss about alcohol is just a fad. People have drunk for years and no one he knows has died from it.
- He is a bit concerned about whether he is safe to drive in the morning, and he doesn't want to lose his licence.
- He thinks the pain could be treated by a tablet, which is what he wants.
- He does not think it is serious, just an irritation.

Cues

What verbal cues will the patient give?

'I know I drink a bit, but all my friends do.'

'If my boss found out how I am in the morning, he'd probably give me the boot.'

What non-verbal cues will the patient give?

- Really not too concerned.
- He really thinks all this fuss about alcohol is a fuss about nothing, and that he is not at risk.
- If alcohol and its consequences are mentioned, he will become concerned.
- He wants to stay healthy.

Psychosocial

- Recent stresses: split with wife and lost his house a year ago.
- Now living back with mum.
- Works as taxi driver – sometimes feels should not be driving early morning as has hangover.
- No significant family history.
- Smoker of 20 cigarettes per day for 10 years.
- No history of drugs.
- No thoughts of self-harm and does not feel depressed.

Examination

Patient will permit an examination to take place. This will demonstrate some tenderness in the epigastric region.

Management

What will the patient expect in management?

- He expects tablets to make him better.

What will the patient accept in management and how involved will he be?

- If offered medication, he will ask how long it will take to work and how long he needs to take it for after he is better.
- If given advice on drinking in a paternalistic way, he will stay quiet but not take the information on board.
- If his understanding of alcohol and its risks is explored, he will be open to new information and will be willing to consider cutting down.

— He will ask for more information to go and read.
— He thinks he can cut down, but once this is explored he will ask you for advice as to what might help him cut down.
— He will take on board and believe the risks of driving.
▶ He will be happy to come back for a review.
▶ He will not be too sure about discussing his separation and house loss.
▶ He will agree to blood tests if the reasons for them are explained.

What questions will they ask?
▶ Will this cause any long-term damage?
▶ How long does alcohol stay in the blood?
▶ Do I need to come back and see you again?

What will he do if he is unhappy with the management?
▶ He will become quiet.
▶ He will minimise eye contact.
▶ He will continue to think he probably doesn't really have a problem and that the doctor is just making too much of things.
▶ He will just want to get tablets and go.
▶ If tablets are not offered he will ask if it's due to a cost-cutting exercise.
▶ If the doctor then begins, at a later stage, to explore his health understanding he will still be open to new information.

Patient record
Frank Spencer
26 years old
144 Avenue Road

PMH
Acne as a child
Not seen for 6 years
No PMH of note
Vaccines all up-to-date

Medication
Nil

17

Jack West by Vicky Taylor

Telephone consultation with the mother of a child who has a sore throat

Part 1

Name: Jack West
Age: 6
Sex: Male
Ethnicity: White British
BMI: Normal
Special visual features: Jack is at school, so mum telephones instead; she seems a bit rushed and flustered

Presenting problem: Jack has a sore throat
What is the diagnosis or problem when framed? Remote assessment of an unwell child with a sore throat
Curriculum statement: ENT and Facial Problems and Care of Children and Young People

Learning outcomes from curriculum statement:
1 Manage primary contact with patients who have an ENT or facial problem.
2 Demonstrate a thorough knowledge of the scientific backgrounds of symptoms, diagnosis and treatment, particularly with respect to ENT interventions of dubious efficacy.
3 Demonstrate an evidence-based approach to antibiotic prescribing, to prevent the development of resistance.
4 Ensure that parents or carers, children and young people receive information, advice and support to enable them to manage minor illnesses themselves.

What knowledge is needed for this case?
▶ Assessment of the feverish child.
▶ Management of a patient with a sore throat.

What is the current evidence relevant to this case?
http://guidance.nice.org.uk/CG47
www.cks.nhs.uk/feverish_children_risk_assessment#-336024
www.cks.nhs.uk/sore_throat_acute#-326932

Part 2

What are you looking for?

A doctor who can take a good remote history about an unwell 6-year-old boy, ascertaining parental concerns about the illness, level of understanding and hopes for what can be achieved during the consultation. Ability to assess the severity of illness, excluding serious causes and negotiating evidence-based patient-centred management plan, while safety-netting appropriately.

What is needed for a good consultation?

▶ Ability to take a history from a third party and assess the severity of illness.
▶ Ability to decide on the appropriate use of a face-to-face consultation.
▶ Ability to obtain a clear understanding of the parent's ideas, understanding, concerns and expectations from the consultation.
▶ Ability to negotiate an appropriate management plan.

What will an above average registrar do?

An above average registrar will take a focused history, asking appropriate questions to risk assess how unwell Jack is and identify that a face-to-face consultation is not needed. They will explore Mum's understanding about Jack's illness and pick up on her expectation for antibiotics. They will further explore her expectations, addressing psychosocial issues and concerns. They will attempt to assess these problems in the context of Jack and his family. They will discuss these issues with mum and reach a shared management plan, taking account of current best practice. This will include advice about symptomatic management of self-limiting illness. They will also 'safety-net', giving mum information about when it is important to seek medical input in the future. They will clarify mum's understanding about what has been discussed.

What will an average registrar do?

An average registrar take a reasonable history from Jack's mum, covering the present illness, as well as mum's expectations. They will exclude serious illness, but may default to a face-to-face consultation. They will address the issue of antibiotics and reach a shared management plan in an evidence-based way.

What will a below average registrar?

A below average registrar will take a basic history about the current problem, but may not ask enough information to exclude serious illness e.g. dehydrated child unable to tolerate oral fluids. They may default to a face-to-face consultation or reassure inappropriately. They may not elicit mum's expectations, or alternatively may pick up these cues, but become confrontational. The consultation may be very doctor-centred.

Part 3

What will be the opening statement (this is a telephone consultation)?

'Hi, I am calling about Jack, my son. He has a sore throat.'

Describe the presenting problem

▶ Normally fit and well.
▶ Been to the GP only 4 times before in last 5 yrs:
  — Verruca.

— Diarrhoea and vomiting.
— Impetigo.
— Sore throat and earache.

▶ Mum says he has had the 'usual coughs and colds' but says he is usually a well boy.
▶ Jack is at school today, mum felt he was well enough to go.
▶ Sore throat for 2 days.
▶ Not getting worse.
▶ Felt a bit hot last night.
▶ Reluctant to eat as throat hurts, but will have ice cream, yogurts and is drinking lots.
▶ Had one lot of paracetamol.
▶ Passing urine and still playing.
▶ Jack lives with his mum and dad and his 9-year-old sister.
▶ Enjoys school, and was keen to go today as he has an art lesson.
▶ The family are going on holiday in 5 days.

How might this problem be framed?

A child with a sore throat whose mother wants advice.

What questions would you expect the candidate to ask to rule in and out other possible diagnoses? What are the answers to these questions?

Would expect the candidate to assess how unwell Jack is, and if he needs to be seen urgently:

▶ no diarrhoea or vomiting
▶ fluid intake good
▶ no rashes
▶ no other concerns
▶ thinks he was well enough to go to school
▶ is not *ill*
▶ no tonsillitis
▶ does get sore throats now and then
▶ last one a year ago
▶ no allergies
▶ no asthma
▶ general health – good
▶ is OK with ibuprofen and paracetamol
▶ parents don't smoke.

Consider the patient's ideas, concerns and expectations

▶ Mum wants advice and reassurance.
▶ She thinks this is just a sore throat and is not unduly concerned.
▶ Jack has had sore throats before and she has always managed with paracetamol at home. However, the family are going on holiday to Spain next week, and she wonder if antibiotics will make him feel better before then.
▶ She is giving him paracetamol – is there anything else she should be doing?
▶ Although he is fairly well now, how will she know if he gets more unwell and needs to see a doctor whilst they are away?

Cues
What verbal cues will the patient give?
'I just wondered if antibiotics would help or not,'
'I've given him paracetamol, but sometimes his temperature doesn't come down – is there anything else I can try?'
'I wouldn't normally phone, its only as we are going away next week.'

What happens if the candidate doesn't pick them up?
When management is discussed, mum will ask 'Will antibiotics be any good?'

What non-verbal cues will the patient give?
Mum will sound a bit flustered.
She has just got in from getting travel money for next week.
She is calm, and seems happy Jack is well.
Not overly concerned or anxious.

Psychosocial
▶ Jack lives with mum, dad and sibling who is 2 years older.
▶ Attends school full time.
▶ Doing well.
▶ Generally active.
▶ Mum works for the Inland Revenue.
▶ Dad is in export business.

Management
What will the patient expect in management?
▶ To have her ideas and queries regarding antibiotics listened to.
▶ For an explanation of what the doctor thinks is going on and why.
▶ Advice regarding managing Jack's symptoms, and when to seek help in future.
▶ Will listen attentively when discussing antibiotics versus symptomatic management.
▶ If concerns are addressed and reasonable explanations given mum will be calm and happy with explanation.
▶ If concerns not addressed and no good reasons are given, patient will firmly ask for child to be seen.

What questions will they ask?
▶ When should I get worried?
▶ Is it safe to just keep giving the paracetamol?
▶ Would antibiotics be any good?

What will they do if they are unhappy with the management?
▶ Will sound unhappy, and get angry/confrontational.
▶ Will ask why you are refusing to give her antibiotics.

Patient record
Jack West
6 years old
98 Grassmarket

PMH
Vaccines up to date
Sore throat and earache 6 months ago
Verruca 8 months ago
Diarrhoea and vomiting 1 year ago
Impetigo 2 years ago

Medication
Nil

18

Lucy Waters by Kafayat Lee

Consultation with a 25-year-old lady with a skin problem
Part 1

Name: Lucy Waters
Age: 25
Sex: Female
Ethnicity: Any
BMI: about 23
Special visual features: Well-dressed, with clothing to cover chest and back, well-made-up

Presenting problem: Has been using topical treatment for her acne but it is not working.
What is the diagnosis or problem when framed? Moderately severe acne, not responding to topical treatment
Curriculum statement: Skin problems

Learning outcomes from curriculum statement:
1   Manage primary contact with patients who have a skin problem.
2   Appreciate the importance of the social and psychological impact of skin problems on the patient's quality of life, including, for example, the effects of disfigurement or sleep deprivation as a result of itching.
3   Recognise how disfigurement and cosmetic skin changes fundamentally affect patient's confidence, mood and interpersonal relationships.
4   Recognise the risk of inappropriate referrals and under-referral.

What knowledge is needed for this case?
▶   Treatment of acne.

What is the current evidence relevant to this case?
▶   Topical treatments, e.g. benzoyl peroxide, retinoid, topical antibiotic.
▶   Oral antibiotics, e.g. lymecycline, erythromycin.

Where can the evidence be found?
www.dermnetnz.org/acne/acne-vulgaris.html
www.cks.nhs.uk/acne_vulgaris

Part 2

What are you looking for?

A focused, patient-centred history, identification of the patient's ideas, concerns and expectations, appropriate advice given to the patient in a patient-centred way, shared management with patient and appropriate and realistic timescales for treatment.

What is needed for a good consultation?

▶ A focused history from the patient, excluding possible triggers and exacerbators of acne.
▶ Identification of the impact of the problem on the patient's life and her hopes for the consultation.
▶ Development of an appropriate shared management plan, avoiding referral at this stage.
▶ Explanation of the treatment options and mechanisms of action in an understandable way.
▶ Safe prescribing and follow-up e.g. contraception advice if given oral antibiotics, and pregnancy advice if given topical retinoids.

What will an above average registrar do?

An above average registrar will take a fluent, focused, patient-centred history from the patient, identifying the patient's relevant past medical history, drug history and current contraception. They will quickly pick up and explore the patient's cues, identifying the patient's thoughts, feelings and concerns about their skin. They will address these concerns giving appropriate information and advice in a patient-centred way. The advice may include: topical benzyl peroxide and/or retinoid; the use of topical or oral antibiotic; advice on condoms if using oral antibiotics for 2 weeks after starting them; option of dermatology referral if she is not happy with the treatment and is finding it psychologically stressful.

What will an average registrar do?

An average registrar will take a reasonable history from the patient, identifying the patient's relevant past medical history and drug history in an organised way. They will explore the patient's cues, identifying the patient's thoughts, feelings and concerns about their skin condition. They will address most of these concerns, giving adequate information and advice in a patient-centred way.

What will a below average registrar do?

A below average registrar will take a poor, unfocused history from the patient. They will fail to identify much of the patient's relevant past medical and drug history. They will fail to pick up or explore the patient's cues, or to identify the patient's thoughts, feelings and concerns about their skin. They will fail to address concerns, giving inadequate information that is not tailored to the patient. They may be very doctor-centred.

Part 3

What will the patient say when they come in?

'I have come about my spots, doctor.'

Describe the presenting problem

- Acne since a teenager, has been getting worse for a few years.
- Much worse in last 6 months.
- Worse just before periods.
- Occasional spots on face, but mainly chest and back.
- Uses oil-free makeup which covers the spots she does get. She knows that oil is bad for her skin and does not use moisturisers, etc. with oil in.
- Has tried topical antibiotic treatment for 7 months with very slight improvement but still is a problem.
- Not been given anything else.
- Uses it every day twice a day.
- Mum puts it on for her.

How might this problem be framed?

Acne – not responding to topical treatment.

What questions would you expect the candidate to ask to try to crystallise what the key problem is and what are the answers?

- Good skin regime – uses Clinique non-comedogenic preparations.
- Has used topical antibiotic treatment with clindamycin for 7 months, some improvement but not as much as expected.
- Non-smoker.
- Half a bottle of wine at weekend.
- No FH of breast, ovarian cancer or thrombo-embolism.
- Currently uses Cilest for contraception. Had used previously for period regulation.
  - Periods have been every 21–35 days since they started, now regular on the pill.
  - No extra body hair and no FH PCOS.
- No significant PMH, no migraines.
- Job been more stressful last few months as Ofsted inspections coming up, but has been coping.
- Not depressed, but the spots do mean that she cannot wear nice clothing.

Consider the patient's ideas, concerns and expectations

- Wants referral to dermatologist.
  - Friend at work has said the dermatologist can give a miracle drug that helps skin.
  - Thinks they can solve the problem in a month.
- Worried that the acne will never go away.
- Worried her boyfriend will leave her.
- Knows about acne – was given a leaflet before and knows some 'bugs' and hormones can cause it.
- Expects to be referred at the end of the consultation.

Cues

What verbal cues will the patient give?
'My friend says the tablet will work in a month.'
'My boyfriend is fed up with me.'

What happens if the candidate doesn't pick them up?
The patient will get irritable and ask more questions.
'There must be something we can do?'
'What drug was my friend talking about?'
'Why can't you refer me?'

What non-verbal cues will the patient give?
She will be dressed smartly, talk reasonably, but will portray an element of desperation that something needs to be done.

Psychosocial
▶ Feels very self-conscious, wonders if her boyfriend will leave her.
  — Have been going out for 6 months.
  — Met at work, and really likes him.
  — Have been sleeping together for 2 months.
▶ Has been on the pill for 3 years to regulate periods.
▶ Wears clothes to cover her chest and back.
▶ Boyfriend frustrated as she has been refusing to go out for the last couple of months as the spots are so bad.
▶ Says he understands, and is supportive, but would like her to feel better about herself.
▶ Works as teacher at the local primary school.

> **Examination card**
> *Lucy Waters*
> Multiple comedones
> 15 pustules on chest
> 10 pustules on back
> Few comedones on face
> No scarring
> No nodules
> No cysts

Management
What will the patient expect in management?
▶ She will expect the doctor to tell her about her options and for a referral to be made at the end.

What will the patient accept in management?
▶ If explained in a reasonable manner, will ask what the doctor recommends and why.
▶ Will be happy to accept a new topical treatment and oral antibiotics if these are explained properly.
▶ Will want a definite review date.
▶ If not explained will request referral to see specialist.

How involved will they be in the management?

▌ She will ask questions about duration of treatment, be keen to explore other options if it means that a referral can still be done if they do not work. She will not want to change her contraception as she is very happy with what she is on.

What questions will they ask?

▌ Cue questions if not picked up.
▌ How does the medication work?
▌ How effective is it?
▌ What happens if it doesn't work?
▌ How long will it take to work?
▌ What would you suggest? Why?
▌ Can I use the treatment if I am on the pill?
▌ When do I come back to see you?

What will they do if they are unhappy with the management?

▌ She will accept what is said but will plan to see another doctor.

Patient record
Lucy Waters
25 years old
7 Grassmarket

PMH
On pill Cilest for 3 years
BP 90/60 taken 2 months ago
Smear taken 2 months ago: normal
No past medical history of note
BMI 23 taken 2 months ago

Medication
Topical clindamycin for acne for seven months

19

Aisha Makda by Keshdip Hayer

Consultation with a lady with a familial genetic problem
Part 1
Name: Aisha Makda
Age: 33
Sex: Female
Ethnicity: Pakistani
BMI: about 20
Special visual features: In Asian-style clothing with a headscarf; fluent English, British born.

Presenting problem: Family history of haemophilia
What is the diagnosis or problem when framed? Family history of haemophilia in a family with a history of consanguinity in marriage
Curriculum statement: Genetics in primary care

Learning outcomes from curriculum statement:
1 Describe how to use family history and knowledge of inheritance patterns to identify those patients in the practice population with, or at risk of, a genetic condition.
2 Describe where to obtain specialist help and advice on inherited conditions.
3 Communicate information about genetics in a comprehensible way, helping patients to make informed decisions and choices about their care.
4 Describe how to take and interpret a family history. This involves:
   — knowledge of relevant questions
   — knowledge of basic inheritance patterns.

What knowledge is needed for this case?
▶ Knowledge of haemophilia and its possible model of inheritance.
▶ Knowledge of how and where to refer.

What is the current evidence relevant to this case?
▶ Haemophilia x linked condition.
▶ Consanguinity increases rate of genetic abnormality.

Where can the evidence be found?
www.bshg.org.uk/genetic_centres/uk_genetic_centres.htm
www.haemophiliacare.co.uk/general/basic_genetics.html

www.library.nhs.uk/GENETICCONDITIONS/SearchResults.aspx?tabID=288 &catID
=7873

www.library.nhs.uk/geneticconditions/viewresource.aspx?resID=148497&tabID=288
&catID=7776

Part 2

What are you looking for?

A candidate who identifies the reasons why the patient has presented and her concern about consanguinity, who explores the patient's understanding and values, and who shares correct information with the patient, negotiating a shared management plan. While a basic understanding of haemophilia is needed, an in-depth understanding of haemophilia or genetic problems caused by consanguinity is not required.

What is needed for a good consultation?

- A focused history.
- Awareness of the diversity issues raised in the consultation.
- Ascertaining of the patient's views on termination.
- A negotiated management plan.
- A basic explanation of the sex-linked nature of haemophilia.

What will an above average registrar do?

An above average registrar will take a focused history of the patient's presenting problem, identifying her concern about consanguinity and her need for information on haemophilia and its mode of inheritance. They will identify her willingness to have preconception screening and her unwillingness to consider a termination. They will develop a mutually agreed management plan and will respond to her questions in a patient-centred way. This will ideally include a referral to a geneticist. They will give an explanation of genetic inheritance of haemophilia in an understandable way and will address the issues raised by parental consanguinity sensitively and non-judgementally.

What will an average registrar do?

An average registrar will take a reasonable history, identifying why the patient has come. They will identify some of her concerns and develop an appropriate shared management plan. They may be uncertain how to manage the problem but they will share this uncertainty. They may refer to a geneticist or a haematologist, or may plan to find more information and review the patient. They will give the patient a basic understanding of haemophilia. They may fail to address issues raised by parental consanguinity. They will do all of this in an organised patient-centred way.

What will a below average registrar do?

A below average registrar will take an unfocused or disorganised history, failing to understand why the patient has come. They will superficially explore the patient's ICE and will make assumptions about the patient's views on screening, termination and children with special needs. They will fail to explain haemophilia, or will do this incorrectly or in a poorly understandable way. The consultation may be disorganised and doctor-centred. Management plan may be inappropriate or unfocused.

Part 3

What will the patient say when they come in?

'Hello, I just wanted some advice. My husband and I are thinking of having a baby in a few years but there may be a problem.'

Describe the presenting problem

▶ Patient opens a piece of paper with 'haemophilia' written on it.
▶ Two nephews on her side of the family have haemophilia: one is aged 2 and the other aged 1.
▶ The 2-year-old nephew belongs to her 28-year-old sister, who also has a 6-year-old girl who is fit and well. This sister lives in New York.
▶ The other nephew is the only child of her 26-year-old sister and he is on injections. It was this sister who advised her to see the doctor. She lives in Canada.

How might this problem be framed?

Family history of haemophilia in a patient considering having a baby, where consanguinity may also be an issue.

What questions would you expect the candidate to ask to try to crystallise what the key problem is and what are the answers?

▶ Both your sisters have married first cousins, but you have married outside the family. Your sisters have married sons of your mother's sister.
▶ There are no other genetic problems in the family as far as you are aware *but* your parents are also first cousins.
▶ Both your sisters' husbands seem well.
▶ You are not planning on starting a family in the immediate future.
▶ You have an Implanon in place and it serves you well.
▶ You would never contemplate an abortion. It is against your faith, but you also think it is wrong. Life begins at conception.

Consider the patient's ideas, concerns and expectations

▶ You know marrying in the family can be a problem but don't know why. You think problems are more likely but don't know what that means.
▶ You don't know much about haemophilia.
▶ You don't know much about other genetic problems.
▶ You have not been on the internet. You came to the doctor to find out more.
▶ You think the doctor will give you information on haemophilia and the chances of your child having this.
▶ You don't expect the doctor to look at other possible genetic problems.
▶ You have a positive view of children with disability but would obviously like to prevent illness if possible.
▶ You are not desperate for a child but would like one at some point.
▶ You are a bit concerned because your parents wanted you to marry in the family, and you didn't. Although they accept your husband, you are a bit worried about what they might say if you have a child with special needs.
▶ You do not want to look at other aspects of preconception care today.

Cues
What verbal cues will the patient give?
'My parents are first cousins' is to be dropped as a cue. Information on this only given if doctor asks directly about other consanguinity in the family or picks up on the cue. This is not essential to 'pass' the case.

Otherwise patient is very up front with all the information she has, and with her concerns.

What non-verbal cues will the patient give?
Confident, matter-of-fact, just wanting information.

Psychosocial
- Happily married for 2 years to a businessman aged 25.
- Not really an arranged marriage, but was a friend of the family.
- Non-smoker.
- Non-drinker.
- Muslim background but not very active.

Examination
No examination is needed.

Management
What will the patient expect in management?
- Information on haemophilia and how it is inherited.
- Advice on what she needs to do if planning a pregnancy.
- Possible identification of issues raised by parental consanguinity.

What will the patient accept in management?
- An explanation of what the doctor thinks needs to be done and why.
- Once she is told about the likely inheritance pattern she will want to know if she can be screened to see if she is a carrier.
- She will be happy for her GP to do this, but if offered a specialist referral will be very willing to be seen.
- She doesn't think she can get much more information from her sister, but if asked to find out more she will say she will try, but will ask what else can be done at the moment.
- Her eldest sister does not seem to be coping well at the moment, and her other sister is 12 weeks pregnant and feeling pretty unwell with morning sickness.
- If the doctor identifies possible issues raised by parental consanguinity, she will be grateful he has raised it as she hasn't really thought of this.
- She will be happy to have a blood test

How involved will they be in the management?
- Will ask questions to clarify.

What questions will they ask?
- What tests can be done?
- What do the tests look for?

> ▶ What happens if the tests are positive?
> ▶ What can be done?

What will they do if they are unhappy with the management?
▶ Will ask where she can get more information.

Patient record
Aisha Makda
33 years old
25 Larkrise

PMH
Implanon put in 2 years ago
Nil else of note

Medication
Nil

SH
Non-smoker
BMI 20
No alcohol
BP 118/76 taken 2 years ago

20

Mukul Bhatt by Uma Mahalingappa

Consultation with a gentleman with raised blood lipids

Part 1

Name: Mukul Bhatt
Age: 42
Sex: Male
Ethnicity: Asian
BMI: about 30
Special visual features: Smartly dressed gentleman in a suit and tie

Presenting problem: Hyperlipidaemia management
What is the diagnosis or problem when framed? A patient looking to manage his raised blood lipids
Curriculum statement: Metabolic Problems

Learning outcomes from curriculum statement:

1 Recognise that non-concordance is common for chronic metabolic conditions (e.g. diabetes) and respect the patient's autonomy when negotiating management.
2 Communicate the patient's risk of complications from obesity and diabetes mellitus clearly and effectively in a non-biased manner.
3 Recognise that patients with metabolic problems are frequently asymptomatic or have non-specific symptoms, and that diagnosis is often made by screening or recognising symptom complexes and arranging appropriate investigations.
4 Advise patients appropriately regarding lifestyle interventions for obesity, diabetes mellitus, hyperlipidaemia.
5 Describe the role of particular groups of medication in the management of diabetes (e.g. antiplatelet drugs, angiotensin-converting enzyme inhibitors, angiotensin-II receptor antagonists, and lipid-lowering therapies).

What knowledge is needed for this case?

How to identify, assess and manage someone at high risk of CVD.

What is the current evidence relevant to this case?

Risk factors:

- age
- sex
- smoking status
- systolic BP taken as average of 2 measurements
- total non-fasting cholesterol
- HDL non-fasting cholesterol
- TC:HDL-C ration
- non-fasting glucose
- FH of early CVD
- central obesity of more than 90 cm waist in Asian males
- low HDL, less than 1.0 mmol/L in men
- impaired fasting glucose.

Charts not validated for non-Caucasian patients

Treatment if risk more than 20% in 10 years

- lifestyle
- lipid reduction
- antithrombotic

Cholesterol target of 4.0 mmol/L or 25% reduction, whichever lower

LDL target 2.0 mmol/L, or 30% reduction whichever the lower

Aspirin 75 mg once BP less than 150/90

Where can the evidence be found?

www.bcs.com/download/651/JBS2final.pdf.

Part 2

What are you looking for?

A registrar who can take a good focused history of risk factors for CVD from the patient, identify the reasons behind why the patient has come and his thoughts on his hyperlipidaemia and family history, recognise the patient has a risk of CVD of greater than 20% in 10 years, give appropriate information and convey risk data to the patient in an understandable way, negotiate a shared management plan, bearing in mind the patient's health beliefs.

What is needed for a good consultation?

- A focused history.
- Identification of level of risk of CVD.
- Appropriate choice of examination.
- Addressing of ICE and development of a shared management plan with adequate follow-up.

What will an above average registrar do?

An above average registrar will clarify the reason the patient has come, identifying what has precipitated presentation now. They will establish what has been done previously and what the patient's understanding of hyperlipidaemia is. They will pick up and explore both verbal and non-verbal cues, leading to an understanding of both the family history and the patient's own risk factors of CVD. They will explore risk factors of CVD, identifying that the patient has a risk of over 20% in 10 years.

They will re-check the blood pressure, do a CVS exam and ascertain the patient's weight. They may assess the abdominal circumference. They will explain to the patient the risk of CVD and the need for further investigations, lifestyle changes and medication in an understandable and non-judgemental way, reaching a shared understanding with the patient and developing a negotiated management plan. Follow-up will be appropriate, including blood tests if statins are recommenced.

What will an average registrar do?

An average registrar will clarify the reason the patient has come, identifying risk factors for CVD, and make an assessment of the 10-year risk of an event. They will try to establish what has been done previously and explore the patient's understanding. They will identify the family history although they may not identify the patient's thoughts and fears on this.

They may re-check the blood pressure, do a CVS exam, ascertain the patient's weight and assess the abdominal circumference. They will explain to the patient the risk of CVD and the need for further investigations, lifestyle changes and medication in an understandable and non-judgemental way, reaching a shared understanding with the patient and developing a negotiated management plan. They may prescribe, or may wait till blood tests are back, depending how the management is negotiated. Follow-up will be adequate.

What will a below average registrar do?

A below average registrar will fail to define why the patient is presenting. They will make an incomplete risk assessment from the history and examination and may fail to identify level of risk or investigate further. Exploration of cues and ICE will be cursory. Explanations may be incomplete or difficult to understand and will not fit into the patient's health understanding. Family history will be superficially explored. They may prescribe a statin and aspirin but will take minimal steps to ensure concordance. Follow-up may be inappropriate, disjointed or absent. The consultation may be doctor-centred or disorganised.

Part 3

What will the patient say when they come in?

'Hello. I have come about my recent blood tests.'

Describe the presenting problem

- Wants to discuss his cholesterol.
- Blood tests done a month ago after seeing the practice nurse for his new patient check.
- Has been told by reception his cholesterol is high and he needs to see a doctor.
- Was told all his other tests were fine.
- Was put on simvastatin by his previous GP, who told him that he had to take a tablet for his cholesterol but did not explain why.
- Has not been taking his tablets regularly at all and has run out of them for over a month.
- He is not diabetic or hypertensive.

What diagnoses might relate to this problem?
▶ Hyperlipidaemia.
▶ Raised CVD risk.
▶ Concern about his lipids and the need to discuss them.

What questions would you expect the candidate to ask to try to crystallise what the key problem is and what are the answers?
Only give this information if the doctor asks specifically.
▶ Wasn't fasting at the time of this blood test or the previous one at the other surgery – had not been advised to do so.
▶ Had a cup of tea and some white toast both mornings and had not stopped drinking alcohol before the test was done.
▶ Don't know how high your cholesterol was.
▶ Non-smoker.
▶ Get little exercise – no time.
▶ Diet: tries to eat healthily as you were told this would be good for your cholesterol, but still your wife uses a lot of ghee.
▶ Uncle died at 48 of a heart attack.
▶ Mum and elder brother have hypertension.
▶ Grandfather had a stroke.
▶ Dad has diabetes, has had for 15 years.
▶ Drink one pint of beer most days.
▶ Don't take aspirin.
▶ No chest pain, shortness of breath, etc.
▶ Fit and well.

Consider the patient's ideas, concerns and expectations
If the doctor asks about your concerns:
▶ You don't know much about what high cholesterol means and whether you should be concerned.
▶ You are concerned about your family history.
▶ You want advice.
    — What is high cholesterol?
    — What does it mean for you?
    — Is it because you are overweight or do you need to take the tablets.
    — If so, how long for?
    — Really doesn't want to take tablets long term.
    — Will it come down if you exercise and change your diet further?
    — What else can you do?
▶ You are hoping that you need no medication at all.

Cues
What verbal cues will the patient give?
'But it's only a little high'
'I am fit and well.'

What non-verbal cues will the patient give?
Looks unhappy about taking medication

Reflective and thoughtful
Slowish speech, but not depressed.

What happens if the candidate doesn't pick them up?
The patient will ask more questions.
'But surely my cholesterol is only a little high?'
'But I am fit and well, so what is the point?'

Psychosocial
▶ Married for 20 years.
▶ 2 children, 18 and 16.
▶ Businessman in the area.
▶ Stable job.
▶ Minimal stress.
▶ Wife does all the cooking.

Examination
If an examination is requested, you will ask what the doctor wants to look for and why. You will then give a copy of the examination card below.

Mukul Bhatt
Examination card
BP 120/70
BMI 30
Abdominal circumference 106 cm
No clinical signs of raised cholesterol
CVS exam normal

Management
What will the patient expect and accept in management?
▶ Is pretty sure he doesn't need any medication and hopes this is the case. He wants to have the problem explained to him as he feels that he has little information.
▶ If the doctor suggests he needs more tests he will look surprised and ask why. He will be happy if the doctor explains the other tests are needed to get further fasting results. He will ask when he has to fast from.
▶ If the doctor raises issues about his family history, he will want to know how this is related to his cholesterol levels.
▶ If the doctor suggests he exercise more, he will take this on board.
▶ If the doctor suggests a change in diet, he will indicate that this may be hard, as his wife does all the cooking. If the doctor suggests he see a dietician, he will say he thinks that will be a waste of time as it is his wife who needs to know everything. The kitchen is not his domain. If he is given a diet sheet, he will ask what kind of foods it has on it, indicating that he eats mainly Asian food.
▶ If he is asked to stop alcohol, he will indicate that he only has 5 pints or so a week, indicating a little alcohol must be good for him.
▶ If the doctor asks to put him back on his statins, he will ask why and what other options there are.

▶ If the doctor wants to put him on aspirin he will ask why, and what the side effects are.

How involved will he be in the management?
▶ Will be gently reflective and questioning.
▶ Will ask the doctor whether he should take the tablets now or wait.

What questions will he ask?
▶ He will ask about what he needs to do and why. This process will depend where doctor goes with management, but with each suggestion the doctor gives, he will explore further if given the time.
▶ If the doctor goes into a long monologue with no space for him as a reflective patient to ask questions, he will not push to interrupt.
▶ If then time is given for questions at the end he will indicate that he has several and then one at a time will question the doctor's suggestions, only moving on to the next area after the previous one is finished. If the doctor cuts him off or rushes him, he will not push himself or his questions forward. He needs to be given space and time.
▶ What is high cholesterol and should he be concerned?
▶ What does it mean for him?
▶ Is it because he is overweight or does he need to take the tablets?
▶ If so, how long for?
▶ Will it come down if he exercises and changes his diet further?
▶ What else can he do?
▶ Should he be concerned about his family history?

What will he do if he is unhappy with the management?
▶ Will show that he is unconvinced, and indicate that he will need to think about it.

Patient record
Mukul Bhatt
42 years old
140 Caster Avenue

PMH
Nil of note
Well man check with nurse 1 month ago
BP 140/90
Bloods done:
FBC normal
U and E normal
Fasting glucose 5
Cholesterol 6.9
HDL 0.8
Trig 1.5

Medication
Simvastatin 20 mg once daily 30 tablets
Last issued by previous practice 2 months ago

SH
Non-smoker

21

John Maddison by Caroline Taylor-Walker

Consultation with a 55-year-old gentleman post myocardial infarct
Part 1
Name: John Maddison
Age: 55
Sex: Male
Ethnicity: White British
BMI: Slightly above normal
Special visual features: Slightly rugged, stubble, clean, fleece and jeans

Presenting problem: Routine follow-up post myocardial infarction (MI)
What is the diagnosis or problem when framed? Health promotion and management of a gentleman post MI
Curriculum statement: Healthy people: promoting health and preventing disease

Learning outcomes from curriculum statement:
1 The risk factors for disease including alcohol and substance abuse, accidents, child abuse, diet, exercise, genetics, occupation, social deprivation and sexual behaviour.
2 Change patients' behaviour in health promotion and disease prevention.
3 Demonstrate an understanding of the patient's (and where appropriate the family's) expectations and the community, social and cultural dimensions of their lives.
4 Be able to judge the point at which a patient will be receptive to the concept and the responsibilities of self-care.

What knowledge is needed for this case?
- Secondary prevention of a patient post MI.
- Motivating health behaviour change.

What is the current evidence relevant to this case?
NICE guidelines on secondary prevention of MI:
- lifestyle
- cardiac rehabilitation
- drugs

▶ heart failure
▶ cardiological assessment.

Where can the evidence be found?
www.bmj.com/cgi/content/extract/334/7603/1112
http://guidance.nice.org.uk/CG48

Part 2
What are you looking for?
The registrar should be able to establish why the patient has come, exploring ICE and assessing how the problem has impacted on him. They should be able to pick up on cues, leading to an understanding of the patient's confusion and lostness as to what is happening to him and what he is supposed to be doing. They should be able to explain what is going on and why, and advise appropriately about secondary prevention, while also addressing the patient's ICE. They may decide to do a cardiac examination. They will arrange blood tests and ensure appropriate follow-up.

What is needed for a good consultation?
▶ Review current management.
▶ Recognise that the patient is unsure of what is going on and what he should be doing.
▶ Explore ICE and pick up and explore cues.
▶ Explain in a way that addresses the patient's need for knowledge and ICE in an understandable way.
▶ Investigate appropriately, e.g. U and E, LFT, CK.
▶ Ensure appropriate follow-up.

What will an above average registrar do?
An above average registrar will take a sensitive, patient-centred history, identify the patient's current physical state, explore his thoughts, feelings and the impact of the MI on his life. He will pick up the cues of uncertainty and confusion, and identify the patient's poor understanding of what is going on, addressing this lack of knowledge in a responsive way. He will chunk and check the information so as not to overload the patient with too much information, ensuring adequate follow-up. He will include some advice on lifestyle, medication, cardiac rehabilitation and further investigations, and will arrange for relevant blood tests. He will offer to chase up the patient's ongoing hospital care, including finding out about the angiogram.

What will an average registrar do?
An average registrar will take a patient-centred history, identifying aspects of the patient's current physical health and ICE, exploring the impact of the MI on his life. They will pick up some cues and explore these. He will give appropriate information on health promotion, although this may be too much to take on board at once, or else not enough. He will include some advice on lifestyle, medication, cardiac rehabilitation and further investigations, and will arrange for relevant blood tests, ensuring adequate follow-up.

What will a below average registrar do?

A below average registrar will take a more doctor-centred history and will fail to explore the patient's current health, ICE and cues, or the impact on his life. He will fail to give the patient the wanted information or will do so in a very paternalistic way, possibly using a lot of jargon. Follow-up will be inadequate, and the consultation may be disorganised or unfocused.

Part 3

What will the patient say when they come in?

'Morning, I have come for a repeat prescription of my tablets.'

Describe the presenting problem

- MI 5 weeks ago.
- Central crushing chest pain for 30 minutes. Wife phoned ambulance.
- Admitted to hospital for a week then discharged.
- Had some blood tests and ECGs, and is now awaiting an angiogram and more tests. No date yet.
- Brought in discharge letter a month ago, and has come in as he is running out of tablets.
- On 5 tablets, but not sure what they are for.
- Has not been in since and has had no blood tests done.
- Is coping with tablets OK but does sometimes forget to take them.
- Feeling fine with no more symptoms.
- Has not been back to work and does not know when he can go back.
- Works as an employed carpenter but thinks work will be too much for him at the moment.
- He thinks he cannot go back till after he has had the test.
- Not really had much explained to him.
- A bit concerned and fed up with it all.
- Not too sure what he should be doing.

What diagnoses might relate to this problem?

- Post MI secondary prevention treatment and concordance.

What questions would you expect the candidate to ask to rule in and out other possible diagnoses?

- He has been fed up since the MI.
- Concerned as dad died of one aged 60.
- Has been told to lose weight, change diet, get exercise, and take tablets, but has not been told why.
- Not too sure what to eat or why, although presumes chips are bad and has cut down on these, as he knows fats are bad for you.
- Has white toast, jam and butter for breakfast.
- Tea with two sugars.
- A cheese sandwich for lunch.
- Meat and two vegetables for tea.
- Couple of pints 5 or 6 times a week.
- Doesn't have fish as it is expensive.

▶ Has never been on a diet.

▶ Has never smoked.

▶ Has been taking the tablets, but does miss some. Has taken his aspirin every day though as he has heard that this is good.

▶ Has been scared to have sex, and this has impacted on his relationship.

▶ Sleep OK, not worrying, and not depressed – just fed up and a bit confused.

▶ He is not denying what is going on, hospital was very busy and he was supposed to see a nurse before he left, but she was off sick. He is hoping to see her at the next appointment.

▶ He was told there might be an exercise class but has not heard any more about this.

Consider the patient's ideas, concerns and expectations

▶ Feels like everything is happening around him, and that he has no control any more.

▶ Just feels fed up with being at home and not working.

▶ Would like to go back to work, gradually to see how it goes.

▶ He doesn't drive so this isn't an issue.

▶ Has little understanding of what is happening and why.

▶ He feels confused and a bit frightened it may happen again.

▶ He is only expecting a repeat prescription initially, but would really appreciate someone taking the time to explain things to him.

Cues

What verbal cues will the patient give?

'I'm not too sure what I am supposed to be doing.'

'I am still not sure what has happened'.

'I don't know what the tests are for, or what they will do.'

'My wife is a lot younger than me.'

What non-verbal cues will the patient give?

Lost and confused in appearance and tone.

What happens if the candidate doesn't pick them up?

Will be repeated several times in different ways, but not turned into questions.

Psychosocial

▶ 2 children from a previous marriage.

▶ Lives with new wife who is 30.

▶ She leads an active life.

▶ Concerned about sex life – can get an erection but just feels tired and no interest at the moment, and a bit scared that it might cause another heart attack. He has not told his wife this.

▶ Works as a carpenter, and is on sick leave.

▶ Been with the company for a while, and is known as a good worker.

Examination

If an examination is requested, he will ask what the doctor wants to look at and why. He will then give the following examination card.

```
· · · · · · · · · · · · · · · · · · · · · · · · · · · · · · · · · · · · · · · · · · · · · · · ·
·                                                                                            ·
:   Examination card                                                                        :
·   John Maddison                                                                            ·
:   BP 120/80                                                                                :
·   CVS and RS exam normal                                                                   ·
:                                                                                            :
· · · · · · · · · · · · · · · · · · · · · · · · · · · · · · · · · · · · · · · · · · · · · · · ·
```

Management

What will the patient expect and accept in management?

▶ Patient would like to be told:
  — What has happened and why.
  — What is likely to happen at the hospital.
  — What he needs to do to help himself and how to do it.
  — What the tablets are for and how to take them.
▶ He will be very open to the doctor's suggestions and will interject with questions to get more information from the doctor, for example 'why' and 'how'.
▶ He will be very amenable to what the doctor suggests.
▶ He will not explicitly ask about sex, but will ask about when he is OK to go to back to work and resume normal activities.
▶ He will want to know when to expect to hear from the hospital and when you want to see him again.
▶ Will ask if he needs any blood tests if the doctor doesn't mention this.

Patient record

John Maddison
55 years old
76 The End Road

PMH
No past medical history of note
Letter from hospital received 4 weeks ago
5 weeks ago: ST elevation myocardial infarct
Discharge Medication:
Aspirin 75 mg od
Ramipril 10 mg od
Atenolol 25 mg od
Simvastatin 20 mg od
Discharge Advice:
stop clopidogrel after 1 month
please check bloods
OPA and angiogram to follow.

22

John Griffin by Krishna Pabbaraju

Consultation with a gentleman with a possible malignancy

Part 1

Name: John Griffin
Age: 48
Sex: Male
Ethnicity: Any
BMI: about 24
Special visual features: Casual dress, slightly unkempt, on the way back from work. Tar stains on his fingers. A packet of cigarettes visible in his pocket.

Presenting problem: Haemoptysis follow-up in a gentleman with a family history of bowel cancer
What is the diagnosis or problem when framed? Cancer prevention with primary and secondary prevention strategies
Curriculum statement: Care of People with Cancer and Palliative Care

Learning outcomes from curriculum statement:

1 Knowledge of the epidemiology of major cancers along with risk factors and unhealthy behaviours.
2 Knowledge of the principles and design of primary and secondary screening programmes.
3 Understand the current population trends in the prevalence of risk factors and cancer in the community.
4 The ability to counsel and explain:
   — risk of disease
   — behaviour.

What knowledge is needed for this case?

▶ Assessment of suspected lung cancer.
▶ Screening for bowel cancer.

What is the current evidence relevant to this case?

▶ Risk factors for both lung and bowel cancer.

- Management of persistent haemoptysis in smokers aged 40 or over.
- Evidence for screening for bowel cancer.

Where can the evidence be found?
www.cancer.gov/cancertopics/pdq/prevention/lung/HealthProfessional/page2
www.chestjournal.org/content/123/1_suppl/50S.full
www.nice.org.uk/nicemedia/pdf/CG027fullguideline.pdf
www.cancerscreening.nhs.uk/bowel/publications/bowel-cancer-the-facts.pdf
www.nhshealthquality.org/nhsqis/files/BOWELSC_STNF_FEB07.pdf

Part 2
What are you looking for?
An organised and sensitive exploration of the story of a patient with a possible lung cancer diagnosis, who may also be at higher risk of bowel cancer. The appropriate management of each of these problems.

What is needed for a good consultation?
- A focused history and choice of examination.
- Identification of the problem of the persistent cough and haemoptysis.
- Identification of a change of bowel habit in a gentleman with a family history of bowel cancer.
- Picking up and exploration of cues of concern.
- Sensitive exploration of the family history and bowel and lung cancer risk factors.
- Appropriate referral for an urgent CXR.
- Negotiated appropriate management of a 2-week history of a change of bowel habit in a gentleman with a family history of bowel cancer.
- Appropriate safety-netting.

What will an above average registrar do?
An above average registrar will take a clear and focused history, enquiring about the patient's ideas about the events so far. They will acknowledge and explore the patient's concerns and why he has them. They will elicit the patient's expectations and develop a shared and appropriate management plan, bearing in mind the current guidelines for both possible lung cancer referral and bowel cancer screening. They will acknowledge the uncertainty of the management of the 2-week change in bowel habit. They may give some healthy lifestyle advice or arrange for some blood tests. They will ensure adequate follow-up of both the possible lung cancer, change of bowel habit and bowel screening. They will do all of this in a patient-centred way.

What will an average registrar do?
An average registrar will take a reasonably focused history from the patient, identifying the two main problems. They will explore relevant risk factors, the patient's cues, identifying the patient's thoughts, feelings and concerns about the haemoptysis and bowel cancer. They will develop a safe and appropriate management plan. There may be a degree of doctor-centredness in the management plan and less of a shared understanding in the areas of uncertainty. Suitable follow-up will be defined.

What will a below average registrar do?

A below average registrar will take an unfocused or disorganised history or fail to elicit the patient's thoughts, concerns and expectations. They may omit exploration of the persistent cough, the change in bowel habit or the family history of bowel cancer. Their management plan will be unsafe and may include an inadequate follow-up. They may not have picked up on the cues given, and so may have had them fed back to them as questions later in the consultation. They may be very doctor-centred.

Part 3

What will the patient say when they come in?

'Can you do something about this cough at all?'

Describe the presenting problem

- Works as an electrician.
- Busy job, but struggling to cope with his job.
- Was treated with antibiotics 2 weeks ago after an episode of haemoptysis.
- Better in himself but cough is still there, and he now has loose motions.
- Has thought about stopping smoking. His wife has been nagging him.
- Could not make time to get to the smoking cessation clinic though, as he is self-employed.
- Has been smoking since he was 15, so will be difficult to stop.
- Will consider stopping, but doesn't want to talk about it today.
- When he came last time the cough was dry but had one episode of haemoptysis.
- Thought it was just because he had been coughing so violently that he had burst a blood vessel.
- Has now been coughing for about 4 weeks.
- Has had haemoptysis about 6 or more times since.
- Bright red blood.
- Not productive otherwise.
- No aggravating or relieving factors.
- Coughs on and off most of the day and keeps him awake at night.
- No other symptoms.
- Has not had it before.
- Feels well and has not had a temperature.
- Bowels loose for the last 2 weeks, since had antibiotics.
- Family history of bowel cancer.

How might this problem be framed?

Persistent cough and haemoptysis in a 48-year-old smoker with a family history of bowel cancer, who has had loose stools for the last 2 weeks.

What questions would you expect the candidate to ask to try to crystallise what the key problem is and what are the answers?

- No shortness of breath.
- No pain.
- No wheeze, etc.
- Does not keep pigeons, budgies, parrots or work with hay.
- No one else has had it.

131

- No weight loss.
- Appetite OK.
- Feels well.
- No aches or pains, etc.
- No FH of lung cancer.
- Has never tried to stop smoking.
- Smoked 30 a day for 32 years.
- Secure job and no children.
- Dad died of bowel cancer 3 months ago at the age of 70.
- Paternal cousin died of bowel cancer 2 years ago at the age of 45.
- Since the antibiotics his stool has been much looser. No blood or mucus.

Consider the patient's ideas, concerns and expectations
- Generally quite happy-go-lucky.
- Haemoptysis scared him. Has thought of lung cancer.
- Also worried about bowel cancer, and more so since dad's death.
- He thinks cancer runs in families.
- Wants to be checked out.
- Expects a chest X-ray, and wants advice about the bowel cancer.
- Thinks this may need an X-ray too.

Cues
What verbal cues will the patient give?
'I think I need a check up.'
'I am concerned . . .'
'I have been more concerned since my dad died . . .'

What happens if the candidate doesn't pick them up?
If doctor moves onto requesting to examine the patient without picking up on cues, patient will ask 'I suppose what I really have come to ask for is an X-ray of my chest and of my bowels to make sure there is nothing wrong?'

What non-verbal cues will the patient give?
Coughs throughout the consultation.
Looks anxious.

Psychosocial
- Married no children.
- Stable job, no financial worries.
- Drinks about 6 pints of beer a week.

Examination
If the doctor asks to examine the patient, they will ask what they want to examine and why. They will then hand over the following examination card.

> **Examination findings**
> *John Griffin*
> Chest exam normal
> Peak flow normal
> Abdominal exam normal
> PR normal
> Weight same as a year ago

Management
What will the patient expect in management?
▶ An X-ray of his chest and abdomen.

What will the patient accept in management?
▶ An explanation of what the doctor thinks needs to be done and why.
▶ He will be happy to do whatever the doctor suggests.
▶ He will ensure that cues about his concern about lung and bowel cancer are turned in to questions if the doctor has not explored these earlier.
▶ He will gently explain he doesn't want to talk about smoking cessation today and would rather come back once he has got his cough sorted, and bowels addressed.

How involved will they be in the management?
▶ Will ask questions but will accept the doctor's answers, asking further clarification about why the doctor is choosing to do what he is doing.

What questions will they ask?
▶ Will ask 'Why?' to the doctor's suggestions.
▶ Do I need an X-ray?
▶ Do you think I might have cancer?
▶ What other checks do I need?

What will they do if they are unhappy with the management?
▶ Will be happy with any management.
▶ Will be a bit put out if doctor does not answer his 'why' questions.

Patient record
John Griffin
48 years old
146 Causway Road

PMH
Chest infection with haemoptysis 2 weeks ago
Nil else of note

Medication
Nil

SH
Smokes 30 cigarettes per day
BMI 24
Alcohol 12 units per week
BP 118/76 taken 2 weeks ago

The next steps

23

Reflections on the process

'You're thinking about something, my dear, and that makes you forget to talk.
I can't tell you just now what the moral of that is, but I shall remember it in a
bit.'

'Perhaps it hasn't one,' Alice ventured to remark.

'Tut, tut, child!' said the Duchess. 'Everything's got a moral, if only you can
find it.'

(Alice's Adventures in Wonderland, pp. 95–6)

By the time you read this, you will have encountered many patients who could
have been in the CSA exam, ranging from Robert Davies with testicular pain and
John Bradford with depression to Eva Peterson with headaches. Patients such as
Jane Doe and her menopausal problems, Melissa wanting the pill, Bradley with
haematospermia and Frank with his alcoholic gastritis have each presented you
with different problems of varying complexity. You have covered a telephone call
about young Jack before he goes on holiday and explored management of the
common clinical problem of acne with Lucy. While many of you may never before
have seen a patient with haemophilia, or even discussed it in a consultation, the
conversation with Aisha will have enabled you to develop skills in dealing with
the more unusual aspects of General Practice. Mukul Bhatt has enabled you to
look at hyperlipidaemia and John Maddison has required you to know and apply
up-to-date guidelines in a less than compliant patient. Finally, John Griffin has
presented you with two possibly serious problems with three key clinical areas
that need to be covered in just 10 minutes.

In this chapter we will look at the reflections and learning points identified
from working with four of the cases in this book. The learning points have been
collated from the thoughts of the registrars who developed the cases in Section 2.
The way the learning set used the cases permitted registrars to watch the same
consultation with two or three different doctors. This provided comparative
insights. You may find that many of their thoughts echo with your own reflections
as you have run the cases yourselves. You may identify other areas that are not
mentioned. What the reflections illustrate is the benefit of developing and using
cases in learning sets, and performing in front of one another.

John Bradford

John encouraged a lot of skill development. The registrars found that it was
very difficult to fit everything into 10 minutes, yet key learning themes emerged.
From watching the case, Hannah tells us that John increased her awareness and

understanding of depression in patients who are tired all the time and helped her to explore skills in gathering a lot of data, while still being open and empathetic. It reinforced to her the need to check ICE and the patient's understanding, while emphasising how empathy facilitates information giving. Shamit pointed out how it was useful to see different ways of asking about suicidal intent. Uma and Krishna saw the benefit of picking up cues in understanding the patient's problem further, rather than just 'taking a psych history.'

On consulting with John, Kesh learned more about developing a shared understanding with the patient and about ensuring adequate safety-netting. In the doctor role, Mark noted the need to rule out organic causes of illness, the importance of its social impact, the requirement for a risk assessment and the need for safety-netting, follow-up and time-management skills. Kafa was encouraged to check the patient's understanding of what had been discussed.

In discussion, the group covered the use and abuse of the PHQ9 and HADS and reinforced the need to exclude organic causes of the symptoms. Caroline said how useful she had found it doing a case with others watching.

Lucy Waters

Kafa wrote the case on Lucy and learned the importance of including all relevant evidence in case writing. This enabled the development of a bespoke management plan, taking on board the latest evidence and the patient's views. She found writing a case to fit into 10 minutes a useful challenge, shedding insight on the kind of cases that could appear in the exam.

Those watching consultations with Lucy acknowledged how useful it was seeing different skills being used to explore the social impact of the skin problem and to discover the patient's knowledge and understanding of acne treatment, as well as her views on it. Caroline points out that it was helpful to see which strategies worked and which did not. In this particular case it became obvious, particularly in discussion at the end, that there were varied knowledge gaps in the management of acne that needed to be addressed by those in the learning set.

From consulting with this case, Shamit identified the need for possible ways to explore the impact of acne on Lucy's life, as well as the need to develop a greater personal knowledge base on the use of retinoids and Roaccutane. Dave found it useful to revisit topical and oral treatment for acne. Uma noted the importance of organisation in the consultation and the benefits of checking the patient's background knowledge and understanding before moving on to management. In looking at management, Hannah acknowledged the importance of adequate advice on commencing antibiotics. Krishna pointed out the need to be willing to use the BNF to check any uncertainty about medications and highlighted again the importance of follow-up. Himanshu identified the need for most of the set to learn more about acne and decided to find and read reliable guidelines on acne management.

Kesh and Caroline also reflected on some less tangible aspects of learning: about how they felt the consultation was going. 'You get a feeling,' says Caroline, 'of what things the doctor says feel good, and what feels awkward or not a clear response.'

Jack West

Jack's case was written by Vicky, who learned several things in its development, including the importance of looking at the patient agenda and defining what she would expect to be present in a basic history. She was then able to establish what she would expect a good doctor to offer. On watching the case, she found different people performed in different ways with quite different outcomes.

Hannah pointed out that watching the case emphasised the difficulty in assessing a patient through a proxy and emphasised the importance of ensuring the doctor checks for relevant 'red flag' symptoms specifically, rather than assuming that because Jack is at school he is therefore well. She noted the value in addressing the mother's health beliefs and understanding. Kesh recognised that doctors who kept their explanation simple and who allowed the patient's ICE to lead the consultation tended to have better outcomes. Krishna also remarked on this. Mark noted the difficulty of assessing through a third party, the need to specifically exclude 'red flags' and the importance of basing any discussion with Jack's mum on her prior understanding. In this case, he said, safety-netting was of great importance. Vicky and Caroline also mentioned the importance of not making assumptions about the severity of Jack's illness, without explicitly checking this. Uma identified the importance of confidence and structure in management, a theme also picked up by Shamit who pointed out the need for focus and clarity in the management development and negotiation.

Melissa Smith

Melissa was a patient who seemed to direct registrar learning in many ways, touching on knowledge, skills, attitudes and behaviours. Vicky pointed out the ease with which fact gathering can be inadequate in cases like this, where there is so much to fit into the time. Smoking history and STI risks had been omitted by some. Vicky also saw the importance of picking up on the cues relating to confidentiality. Hannah noted the significance of checking what the patient understands and the problems caused to the doctor by failing to elicit necessary information that the 15-year-old could give. Hannah also highlighted the usefulness of observing the different ways of assessing Gillick competence in practice. Interestingly, Kesh pointed out that the assessment of competence was one area that registrars need to make particularly explicit in the exam situation, which they may do more implicitly in a real consultation. Kesh also recognised the need to be non-judgemental.

Krishna looked at the importance of a doctor's body language, especially when the doctor is caught a bit off guard, and sees a case that he does not commonly see. Fifteen-year-old girls requesting contraception in the real world usually choose to see young female doctors. Krishna also remarked how the patient narrative gave much of her ICE without this being formally inquired about. Himanshu pointed out that there was a lot to cover in 10 minutes and that the need to explore consent and confidentiality issues was facilitated by getting the trust of the patient. It was also helpful, he felt, to have a good knowledge about the 'pill rules', and how to explain them. Caroline found it useful seeing how others were able to share management plans in a patient-centred way, gauging the amount of information given. Kafa also emphasised the need to try not to cram too much information in, but to chunk and check, realising that everything does not need to be done in one consultation. The offer to cover areas in more detail at a later stage may be just what the patient wants.

Issues about excluding child abuse were also seen to be important and Uma saw common ways in which different doctors addressed this. In the discussion, Shamit found it interesting that his willingness to share what he knew about similar cases helped further exploration of what could be done.

Jane Doe

Jane Doe enabled the registrars, almost unanimously, to identify educational needs and knowledge gaps in the area of HRT, particularly in the area of risks and benefits of different approaches. Caroline commented that it was useful to demonstrate the ability to 'to live through a consultation I had no knowledge about' and Shamit pointed out the value of the BNF, but also the importance of being aware of the differential diagnoses of hot flushes. Dave, Uma and Krishna highlighted the need to explore ICE early and pick up on cues. Dave's words perhaps reflect the feeling of the majority: 'I need to do more reading on the topic' and, in Hannah's words, 'I need to be able to explain it.'

Why reflection?

Reflection on cases used and studied in the learning set is ideal to promote and consolidate learning. I have suggested that this reflection is done as part of running a case in the learning set and Box 8.1 gave a template for this. Delayed formal reflection is also useful to help further reinforce the knowledge, skills, attitudes and behaviours covered in the learning set, making you more likely to recall, and encouraging you to apply, what you have learned. The process also provides you with a further record of your learning and planned changes. A form to help structure this further reflection is given in Box 23.1 below. This can also be used to initiate discussions with your trainer or can be added to the e-portfolio as evidence, if you wish.

BOX 23.1 Reflective review form

Reflective review
Name of case:
Date of learning set:
What did I learn from this case?

How am I trying to apply what I have learned?

What else do I need to do to apply what I have learned?

How could I demonstrate this learning in a consultation?

What will my trainer notice that is different about my consultations?

24

Life beyond CSA Land

'I quite agree with you,' said the Duchess; 'and the moral of that is – "Be what you would seem to be" – or if you'd like it put more simply – "Never imagine yourself not to be otherwise than what it might appear to others that what you were or might have been was not otherwise than what you had been would have appeared to them to be otherwise."'

(Alice's Adventures in Wonderland, p. 96)

At the beginning of this book, I took you to the start of the story of *Alice in Wonderland*. The White Rabbit runs past Alice, worried about being late. Alice follows and falls down the rabbit hole. As we read on we find that Alice, placed in a strange new world that works with very different rules to the world she comes from, begins to adapt. Initially disorientated by the number of times she finds herself changing size, she then begins to make this work for her. As she meets a variety of characters who are not 'real' as she understands reality, she develops relationships and works with that unreality. She learns what to say and what not to say.

As you enter the not so bizarre, but still slightly disorientating world of CSA land, you will also, like Alice, encounter different rules. As you experience the feeling of performing in a role play assessed consultation, where you may feel small and disempowered like Alice, you can identify what can help you to feel tall again. As you meet characters who are not real patients, who do not have real clinical signs, who are not being themselves, like Alice you can begin to work with that unreality. And like Alice in the different world of Wonderland, in CSA land you can learn what things are best not said and what things do need to be said, that you may not feel the need to say explicitly in real life General Practice.

Unlike Alice, you are unlikely to meet a Mad Hatter. Mercury poisoning is not that common in the UK today. However, you may meet someone with a psychosis, an iatrogenic disorder or an occupational health problem. A dozy dormouse likewise is unlikely to appear in your consultation room, but a patient who is tired all the time could well consult. While the Queen of Hearts is not a likely patient to turn up in Croydon, throwing her aggressive weight around, a dissatisfied, angry, complaining relative may well do so.

This book has aimed to be the piece of cake that Alice ate to make her taller. It also aimed, in the way it has been put together, to help you understand the world of CSA land and develop the skills to cope with it. By encouraging you to work in learning sets, it has tried to help you develop learning environments where you can gain from each other and practice performing in that new world.

As you continue to prepare for the CSA, I would encourage you to maintain a longer term focus to your learning. In specialist training, you are looking to prepare for a lifetime in General Practice, not just a one-off exam. Alice's time in Wonderland was short and sweet, and after the dream was over she looked forward to 'gather about her other little children, and make their eyes bright and eager with many a strange tale, perhaps even with the dream of Wonderland of long ago . . .'[1]

The chances are you will pass the exam. After two attempts, 95% of candidates pass. Once that is done, maintaining and developing skills in consultations will be part of your ongoing Continued Professional Development and role play is a fantastic tool for doing this. Once you have passed, I would encourage you not to say goodbye to role play, but look to see how you can use it to help you continue to learn as a GP. You may even, like several of my registrars who have passed the CSA, take under your wing other specialist registrars who are facing the CSA challenge and, like Alice, pass on the strange tales and help the next generation of doctors face CSA land with more insight, skills and confidence.

Reference

1 Carroll L. *Alice in Wonderland and Through the Looking Glass*. London: Pan Books; 1947. p. 134.

Index

abdominal pain 97–100
acne, severe 107–11, 138
Agenda-Led Outcome Based Analysis (ALOBA) 49
alcoholic gastritis 97–101
The Anxious Patient model (Bendix) 10

bowel cancer 129–34
Bradford, John (patient with depression) 72–7, 137–8

Calgary–Cambridge model (1998) 11–12
cancer, suspected malignancies 129–34
case examples
    abdominal pain with substance abuse problems 97–101
    alcoholic gastritis 97–101
    changes to a mole 58–63
    contraception advice 89–92, 139–40
    familial genetic problems 112–16
    haematospermia 93–6
    headaches and migraine 78–82
    hyperlipidaemia management 117–23
    lung and bowel cancer 129–34
    malignancies 129–34
    menopausal symptoms 83–8, 140
    post-myocardial infarct advice 124–8
    pre-conception care 52–7
    severe acne 107–11, 138
    sore throat infections 102–5, 139
    testicular pain 67–71
    tiredness all the time, TATT 72–7, 137–8
case feedback 21–2, 49–51
case preparation
    implementation stages 44–8
    use of writing templates 40–4
    writing own presentations advice 39–48
case reflections 137–42
childhood complaints, sore throat infections 102–5, 139
cholesterol management 117–23
clinical management skills 13, 15–16
competence domains 34
consanguineous relationships, inherited conditions 112–16
consultation skill models 8–12
    suitability for CSA 12–16
contraception advice 89–92, 139–40
CSA exam 3–7
    key domains 13
    learning outcomes 4–5
    pass rates 142
    personal accounts and experiences 24–32
    possible case types 5
    preparation advice 18–23
    writing own cases 39–48
curriculum see GP curriculum

data gathering skills 13, 15
depression, tiredness presentations 72–7, 137–8
diagnosis making 47–8
Disease-Illness model (McWhinney 1986) 10–11
The Doctor, his Patient and the Illness (Balint 1957) 9
domains of Good Medical Practice 34

ENT problems, sore throat infections 102–5
epididymo-orchitis 67–71

exam advice *see* CSA exam; preparing for the CSA
The exceptional potential in each primary care consultation model (Stott and Davis 1979) 9

familial genetic problems 112–16
feedback on cases 49–51
  forms 51
  as learning tool 21–2
The Future General Practitioner (RCGP 1972) 9

genetic problems 112–16
Gillick competency 89–92, 139–40
GP curriculum 33–8
  core competence domains 34
  domains of good practice 34
  interpretative statements 34–5
  practical application exercises 36–8
  use of *The Teaching and Learning Guide* (RCGP) 33–4

haemophilia, consanguineous relationships 112–16
Hayer, Keshdip 31
  case presentation (familial genetic problems) 112–16
headache problems 78–82
health promotion, post myocardial infarct advice 124–8
Helman's folk model (Helman 1981) 10
HRT advice 83–8, 140
hyperlipidaemia 117–23

ICE (patient's ideas, concerns and expectations) 47
inherited conditions 112–16
The Inner Consultation model (Neighbour 1987) 11
interpersonal skills 13, 16
interpretive statements 34–5

Jonnalagadda, Shiloh Jacintha 27
  case presentation (man with haematospermia) 93–6

Kalla, Shamit 26–7
  case presentation (women who is experiencing headaches) 78–82
Kolb's learning circle 20
Kunda, Hannah 25–6
  case presentation (man who is tired all the time, TATT) 72–7

learning outcomes 34–5
  case example 37–8
learning sets 20–3
learning skills 20–2
Lee, Kafayat 29
  case presentation (severe acne) 107–11, 138
Leicester Assessment Package (LAP) 12
lifestyle advice
  hyperlipidaemia management 117–23
  post myocardial infarct 124–8
  pre-conception care 52–7
lung cancer 129–34

Mahalingappa, Uma 30
  case study (hyperlipidaemia management) 117–23
malignancy conditions 129–34
management plans 48
melanoma concerns, mole changes 58–63
menopausal symptoms 83–8, 140
mental health problems, depression presentations 72–7
metabolic problems, hyperlipidaemia management 117–23
migraine presentations 78–82
mole changes 58–63
myocardial infarct 124–8

Pabbaraju, Krishna 32
  case presentation (possible malignancies) 129–34
patient profiles 46
  see also ICE (patient's ideas, concerns and expectations)
peer support, exam preparation 19–23
performance levels and expectations 46

personal accounts and experiences (CSA exam) 24–32
pre-conception care, case writing examples 52–7
pregnancy, pre-conception care 52–7
preparing for the CSA 18–23
    personal accounts 24–32

reflections on the process 137–40

semen, blood discharges 93–6
The seven tasks of the consultation model (Pendleton, *et al.* 1984) 11, 49
sexual health
    contraception advice 89–92
    haematospermia 93–6
Shaffu, Mark 27–8
    case presentation (man with abdominal pain) 97–100
Sharma, Dave 30–1
    case presentation (contraception advice) 89–92, 139–40
Shekhar, Himanshu 26
Six Category Intervention Analysis model (Heron 1975) 10
Six phases of the consultation model (Byrne and Long 1976) 10
skin conditions
    mole changes 58–63
    severe acne 107–11, 138
Smith, Melissa (patient seeking contraceptive advice) 89–92, 139–40
sore throat infections 102–5
substance abuse problems, alcoholic gastritis 97–101

Taylor-Walker, Caroline 29–30
    case presentation (post-myocardial infarct advice) 124–8
Taylor, Vicky 28–9
    case presentation (childhood sore throats) 102–5, 139
The Teaching and Learning Guide (RCGP) 33–4
teenagers, contraception advice 89–92
testicular pain 67–71
timing, of feedback 49–50

tiredness all the time (TATT), student case presentation 72–7, 137–8
Transactional Analysis (Berne 1964) 9

Waters, Lucy (patient with severe acne) 107–11, 138
Webb, Deborah 24–5
    case presentation (testicular pain) 67–71
West, Jack, (child with a sore throat) 102–5, 139
women's health
    contraception advice 89–92, 139–40
    menopausal symptoms 83–8
    pre-conception care 52–7
writing own cases 39–48
    basic templates 40–4
    case example-1 (pre-conception care) 52–7
    case example-2 (skin problems /mole changes) 58–63
    student examples
        case example-3 (testicular pain) 67–71
        case example-4 (tiredness all the time, TATT) 72–7, 137–8
        case example-5 (woman who is having headaches) 78–82
        case example-6 (menopausal symptoms) 83–8, 140
        case example-7 (contraception advice) 89–92
        case example-8 (haematospermia/ blood in semen) 92–6
        case example-9 (alcoholic gastritis) 97–101
        case example-10 (sore throat infections) 102–5, 139
        case example-11 (severe acne) 107–11, 138
        case example-12 (familial genetic problems) 112–16
        case example-13 (hyperlipidaemia management) 117–23
        case example-14 (post–myocardial infarct advice) 124–8
        case example-15 (possible malignancies) 129–34